Prostate cancer: Climbing above it

Nine men tell their stories of how they experienced advanced prostate cancer and how they were lifted above it.

Laurence Lepherd
(Editor)

Published in 2013 by
Laurence Lepherd
PO Box 11387
Centenary Heights
Toowoomba, Queensland, Australia

ISBN-10: 1482383527
ISBN-13: 978-1482383522

Foreword

Surviving, or even thriving, through tough times is a human capacity to be admired, and desired. For most of us, the skills and mindset required to manage adversity well are unlikely to be innate, but rather grow with experience. In the face of personal challenge, we typically stumble, mumble, and bumble along for some time before we begin to accept and learn to deal with our altered circumstances.

This collection of stories is of ordinary Australian men, confronting perhaps the biggest challenge of their lives. Diagnosed with advanced prostate cancer, they were forced to confront their own mortality at the same time as they deal with a myriad of physical, emotional and spiritual challenges and adjustments.

Reading through their stories, I was struck by both the level of suffering each man experiences, and as the tenacity of each man as he 'kept going'. I was also struck by the individuality of each story – each one is a unique journey where the common element (having advanced prostate cancer) is played out in very different ways, in very different lives.

It is left to the reader to marvel that each man had the strength and determination to not just keep going, but also to find ways to connect with others and continue to live their lives in constructive and positive ways. I know they desired to share their journeys as a way of helping others; in some ways perhaps sharing their experiences helped them to 'make sense' of their own suffering.

The stories challenge the notion that men 'won't talk' about deeply personal matters. The nine courageous men who have shared their experiences in this volume have been prepared to 'put themselves out there', to reveal their vulnerabilities and to talk of matters which have hitherto been unspoken.

This collection of the stories of men with advanced prostate cancer will be of use to clinicians, as well as those with advanced prostate cancer, and those who love them.

Finally, these stories owe much to their collector, Dr Laurie Lepherd. Laurie is a deeply spiritual man, and this collection is just one example of his spirituality in action. He demonstrated passion, a tremendous work ethic and much patience in seeking out men who were prepared to share their stories. He listened, he heard, and he took action. This collection of stories was made possible through his strength and determination to make a difference.

Professor Cath Rogers-Clark
Head, Department of Nursing and Midwifery
University of Southern Queensland
Australia

Preface

These stories were told by nine men who had advanced prostate cancer, that is, their cancer had either spread outside the prostate gland or had metastasised to other parts of their body. They were part of a research project that explored the spirituality of men in this condition where spirituality was broadly described to them as aspects of life that lifted them above the ordinary, especially their illness, and helped them towards achieving a better peace of mind.

The men's stories in this book show the ebb and flow of their lives during their journey. Their spirituality involved them connecting with a variety of people, a higher power, places and other important aspects of their lives. These were the things that help them towards a peace of mind that made life more manageable for them and their wives, partners and families.

Each of these stories is unique; they reflect the individuality of the participants. They not only show how challenging life is to men who have advanced prostate cancer, but they show how each man was frequently creative in the way he tried to cope so that his life continued to have value. Apart from minor editing, I have left their language style as they spoke rather than edit it to make it a grammatically correct written story. I believe this conveys a little more of each man's character.

It is hoped that men with prostate cancer reading this book will find something helpful for them during their own journey. While the stories were from men with advanced prostate cancer, observations from other men whose prostate cancer was at an earlier stage indicated that there were some commonalities with their own journey. They will probably see elements of themselves in the men's stories and to this extent, may realise that they are not alone as they face the challenges in front of them. As one of the men said about his illness: "I'm going to climb above it!".

Laurence Lepherd
Toowoomba, Queensland, Australia
January 2013

Contents

The men's stories

Michael[1]

Michael was spending all the time and energy that he had in educating others about prostate cancer and its issues. Michael was 64 at the time of the interview.

Beginnings

Well I guess the best place to start is at the beginning and it goes back to the first indication that something was wrong was on Easter Monday '08 when I had severe pain across my lower back, buttock region and in my right side at 2 or 3 in the morning. It eventually eased off and I went to see the on-call doctor at my local medical practice in Cairns and, after about a half-an-hour examination he diagnosed it as acute sciatica. I went to see my own GP and he confirmed the diagnosis after another thorough examination.

Unfortunately, after 2 to 3 months there was no real improvement in the pain. My GP got on to a visiting neurosurgeon and referred me to him. The neurosurgeon was pretty candid about it and said "I don't like the sound of this at all. If I have to operate on your spine there's only a 50-50 chance of success" and he said, "If it goes pear-shaped, you can end up in a wheelchair". I said "Oh, great!" But he said, "However, let's get a bone scan, MRIs and CT scans". All of that was arranged. We saw him again on the 7th of July and he said, "I'm afraid I have good news and bad news. The good news is we know what's causing the sciatic pain. Unfortunately, it's these shadows at the base of your spine". And, Margaret, my wife, who was with me, said "You mean these are secondaries, don't you". He said, "I'm afraid so. We need to find the primary". He said, "I suspect it's prostate cancer but that's not my field. I'll refer you to a urologist in the hospital." We saw him a few days later and he did a digital rectal examination and a PSA and I went back later for a biopsy. My PSA was

---

[1] The names of all men, women and places in this book, except for eminent, international figures, have been changed to protect their privacy.

126. A week later when I had the biopsy it was 138. The biopsy confirmed that I had prostate cancer Stage IV T3 M1+ with a Gleason score of 8.

Shock of diagnosis

The urologist was very candid and said, when we asked him about it, I had a life expectancy of three to four years; maybe a bit less, maybe a bit more. He said, "We will have a cure for it one day, but you're not going to live to see it and you've got to look at it as bringing forward your retirement age by 20 years". I was given two choices of treatment: 1) surgical castration or hormone therapy treatment. Other treatments were not suitable as the cancer was not clearly defined and had left the prostate and surrounding areas and had travelled to my skeleton. The first medication was a tablet called Cosudex, to bring the PSA under some sort of control, and then a slow-release implant injection, Zoladex, which lasts three months, and my PSA came down. The hormone therapy aims to reduce the testosterone because the testosterone feeds the cancer and it's important to control it.

Seeking a normal life

I carried on working. My background is in the mining industry, specifically explosives, drilling and blasting. I work for myself as an explosives security and safety consultant. We were living a very active life at the time and I had no side-effects. And that's the problem with prostate cancer. There are no uniform real indicators. Everybody responds differently and the symptoms are different for everybody. Some have them; some don't. I didn't have any. And, again, similarly with treatment. Everyone responds differently to the treatment. I have hot flushes and also cold flushes, which I think were worse than the hot flushes. You just can't get warm sitting in front of the fire. You try a cup of tea or coffee in the middle of the night. You're frozen. You're not shivering; you are just cold – very cold.

In early March '09 I went for radiotherapy, solely for pain management. My pelvis was riddled with it (the cancer) and it was very uncomfortable to sit on a seat. The secondaries actually were at the base of the spine, thoracic spine, ribs and my right shoulder. However, there may have been other secondaries there but they did not show up in the scans. I think they've got to be bigger than 3 mm to show up. The radiotherapy was for a month and they did, I guess, two thirds of my pelvis and my right shoulder.

Then in September '09 we decided to come back to the Gold Coast for our support network, not for access to better medical treatment but the support network and easier access for my sons. I think it will be better for them as we have no family here in Australia apart from the two boys, one in Brisbane and one in Sydney.

Treatment and side-effect trauma

So, at present, the drugs are still working. My PSA is 0.13. How long that will last is anyone's guess. The side-effects are, I guess, worse than the treatment because I have psoriatic arthritis that makes it very difficult to write. Also, I have osteoporosis so there is medication for both. There's the hormone therapy but one of the common side-effects that hasn't affected me but I'm having treatment for it as the predominantly long bones become very brittle because of the treatment so I have a monthly infusion of Zometa (that places) a scaffolding type structure over the bones to help strengthen them. And that's it.

The treatment I am on is solely for the control of my testosterone because the testosterone feeds the cancer. In time, the tumours will build up a resistance to the drugs and, when that happens, that's it. I have the option of chemotherapy but I haven't quite decided whether I will take that because the side-effects are rubbish!, and the last three months I've been pretty down because of the side-effects from the cancer treatment and from the other drugs – complete loss of energy, very lethargic and not interested in things. I've actually come off one of the drugs – Cosudex, still on the Zoladex, and, whether it's psychosomatic or not, I think I'm marginally better but I'll know next week whether that has made a difference to controlling the cancer. I'm due for a PSA on Monday and will find out if it's risen.

Coping with stress

We've had our ups and downs. I think we've handled it very well. I mean, one of the first things we did when I was first diagnosed was to send over 100 emails out to family, friends, work colleagues and people I've met and told them what had happened to me and quite a few wrote back and said, "Thanks very much for the reminder – we are off to see the doctor for a check-up". A few followed it up and said, "Thanks for saving my life" because they were in fact diagnosed with cancer; they were in the early stage and were successfully treated.

I should also say that Dad had it but didn't die from it; my older brother has prostate cancer and has been successfully treated with radiotherapy. I was having checks done on an annual basis and nothing was picked up. The urologist said to me, "Look, don't beat your head around. That's it. You have a very aggressive cancer". The only absolute definitive test for prostate cancer is a biopsy. Even then, if you don't cover the whole prostatic capsule, you could miss out some areas. And he said, "You could have come in here and I could have done a biopsy and in another six weeks you could have come back here and you would have got it because that's the nature of the cancer you've got". It's very aggressive.

Communicating with others

The life expectancy I was given was three to four years. I was not in a position to stop work. It's not in my make-up to just pull down the blinds and lock the door and wait for the rainy day. As I say, I communicated with other people … to help. That's how I've handled it. I've carried on working to the best of my ability. I no longer do site work so my income has been slashed. Fortunately, we have income protection, otherwise we'd be in Queer Street. I've always given something back to the community. I've been in Rotary off and on since the '70s in Singleton in the Hunter Valley, and I've been in Lions as well. In January 2010 I became a Prostate Cancer Foundation of Australia (PCFA) Ambassador and that helped me cope with it. I go around to industry groups, service clubs talking about prostate cancer to raise the awareness of prostate cancer among Australians. I always say, especially in industry groups, that female employees should come along as well so they can pass the information along to their husbands, partners, brothers, fathers, uncles etc … So that's how I cope. I'm not a religious person.

It doesn't fully go away. It's there all the time. I get on with my work. I do a little bit of administrative work for a client in Tasmania when I feel like it. I'd be lucky recently if I did one or two hours a week.

Life experience – a traveller

If you asked me what sort of person I am, I would say I am a travelling man. By that I mean that in my working career in contract blasting, explosive manufacturing etc I've travelled around the world – Africa, Middle East, Asia, Australia, Europe – I have seen abject poverty and people struggling to make a crust and yet they give hundreds of dollars to the church but they don't still get anything back in return. Yes, they can give help to some people but overall, for the world-wide community, I don't think they do a great deal. I've had a great life. I've always given something back to the community. That's why I'm an ambassador. People say, "why do you talk about it?" If I talk to a hundred people and save one life, it's worth it.

Climbing above it

Cancer changes you; I don't know whether it (my spirituality) does or not. It may have fluctuated a little bit, I suppose, in that I suffered from depression – and there have been days that I have, without question. I'm not going to let it get me down. I'm going to climb above it.

Getting on to being an ambassador – people say, "why do you do it?" Well, I'm giving something back to the community. I'm helping people that are perhaps less fortunate than me. And people will listen to somebody who has travelled the journey and they'll get something out of it, even if it's the wives nagging "well, go and see the doctor". I mean, the key message really, particularly for men, is that they should listen to their body. If they have a pain in their body, it doesn't matter where it is, they should go and see a doctor. It means there is something wrong with them. I try to relate that to them owning an expensive car, boat, piece of plant or equipment. They value it and look after it. A lot of men in today's western society don't look after themselves. I think that's the key message. We've got to try to change that attitude. We've got to try and help ourselves by looking after ourselves.

Support of friends

I don't think I need more spiritual support personally. I mean, we have a good bunch of friends around. If I'm asked how I feel, I normally get into trouble from Margaret when I say "I'm fine", and she says, "You're not fine", and of course it's only Margaret that sees the ups and downs and there are some days I'll be physically down; I'll be ashen. And that can last for a few hours; it can last all day.

When someone has a terminal illness, they expect you to be losing weight, being withdrawn and so on and so forth. I've put on a little bit of weight, but that's the drugs, and normally my colour's pretty good.

Breakdown in the medical support system

I mean, talking about support, this is where the whole system (and this is not so much spiritual support but medical-type support), for people diagnosed with advanced prostate cancer, you've got to go out and find it all yourself, and that's no disrespect to the medical specialists and the GP. They have to be educated themselves. And this is where the PCFA agents have got to do a lot more in putting together booklets for specialists and GPs and giving the GPs more information about prostate cancer support groups. It's that type of thing that I want to raise with the PCFA – I mean, they are aware of that and they are starting to do it. They've got a teleconference this Thursday and I've already put a lot of these issues on the agenda. The biggest gap is that there is no case manager for somebody diagnosed with a terminal illness. I mean, I have other illnesses as well which I'll talk about to highlight what pings us off. I've got Essential Tremor, Coxsackie B4, I've got ulcerated colitis, I've got psoriasis, psoriatic arthritis and osteoporosis. Do the doctors communicate with each other about these things? No. You've got to tell them to send the results of the various tests to each other. I think it's crazy. You're the one that's sick but you're reminding the doctors to do what I think is part of their responsibility, because, if somebody is diagnosed for one of my conditions, you don't know what the impact is on another one – maybe yes, maybe no.

In industry, if there is a major workplace accident, someone is appointed to facilitate an investigation. It's a case. I believe that the absence of such a provision for medical issues is a big, big gap that makes it much harder for people with a terminal illness.

My working career has been associated with contract blasting and explosive manufacturing. In twenty years now I've been in occupational health and safety in the explosive mining industry. Now, I firmly believe that everybody has a right to come home from work in the way they went to work. To be a Loss Control Practitioner, you've got to have a hard head, and you've got to be prepared to beat it against a brick wall, until the management of a company change their way of doing things. We're talking about the lack of indirect medical support; it's not there. So if I can help in change, then it's been worthwhile.

Leaving a mark

Women talk about their health issues. Men don't. The example I use is breast cancer. There is only one national group for prostate cancer. There are 33 groups – which is crazy as far as I'm concerned – for breast cancer. In the end, there's a lot of money being wasted on administrative duties whereas, if there were one or two for breast cancer, perhaps they would be much further ahead. If I can encourage men to go to the doctor, look after themselves on a regular basis, then it has not been in vain in getting prostate cancer. Sure, it's still going to be hard on the family and everything else, but perhaps I'll have left a mark somewhere.

I'd like to raise the awareness of men and their partners. They have to ask questions and, if they don't get satisfactory answers, they've got to get them somewhere else. GPs and urologists and, to a lesser extent, pathologists have to be far more candid and frank with their patients. Quite a few people were not given correct information about their treatments and side-effects and this has resulted in the breakdown of the marriage. They weren't told that their loss of libido was going to happen. Suddenly they find out the hard way. And that really pings me off. I won't say they are not doing their job but the PCFA has to get some guidelines out to the specialists and doctors. My wife, Margaret, has been with me all the way and her career as a nurse and nurse educator has been extremely beneficial when talking to the medicos, and asking questions in a different way. This helps us better understand the answer.

Craig

I arrived at Craig's home after about three hours of travel and was warmly welcomed by both Craig and his wife, Dianne. Craig was unsettled during the interview because of the medication he was taking and some parts of the narrative show this. At the time of the interview, Craig was 79.

Spirituality – early days

I was brought up Church of England. I started writing a story of my life and got up to quite a few hundred pages. A few years ago I stopped doing it. For some reason I could not start again. I could type 30 words a minute but now I can't type one word a minute. I was a choir boy; I went to High Church of England and my mother said, for school, Sunday school and church, "You can do anything you like, you two boys; you can lie on the ground, kick, say you're sick, but you'll go to school every day and you'll go to church on Sunday." Although, when I was aged 14, I was given a choice.

I actually found a good Sunday School at Waterford. My dad bought a nice home there, and I went there because I respected Mr Molton who was the lay preacher. We went there a while ago and we found a little plaque at the front saying that the foundations were laid in his memory. We painted the roof of the church and we did it because we all liked him. Then, I went my own way, was married and had a couple of children.

The start of prostate cancer – "the worst ..."

I was finding it very difficult to void in 1993. I had actually bought a milk run. I was living in Cairns, flew down, saw the broker and saw the books, although you can't really tell from the books. I could have bought a home in Brisbane and a taxi for the price I paid for the milk run, but my wife and I rented a house and did the milk run. After a short time deregulation came in. There was a lot of heart-ache for milk vendors. Before I did that I went to see a doctor and he gave me a clean bill of health. I said that I was going to be working 12 hours a day, seven days a week, and I've got to do that for four solid years. He gave me a full set of tests, sent me to the urologist who did tests; he passed me. Then after a few years I started to void continually. I kept putting off ... I went to see a urologist who in those times was the number one person and he said, "This is the worst ... ah ... the worst ... urethra I've ever had dealings with". I said, "What happens?", and he said "I've got to clean it, repair it". I said, "When?" and he said "NOW, TODAY, YOU'VE GOT TO GO TO HOSPITAL NOW!" I told him what I was doing and he said, "You're going to be stretchered out of here any second". He did the operation.

"Devastated"

I was devastated! Devastated, yeah, devastated, because it's, um ... an attack on your manhood! I was silly enough to be thinking along those lines, and a lot of men do think along those lines, don't they, do you agree?

Yeah, yeah ... so when he did the operation, I was badly burned by the laser so the next day ... talk about agony ... it's a step above agony. I couldn't get out of bed. The sisters and doctors came up and I'd have to show them and my scrotum was about huge and the doctor came and said, "I'm sorry, old chappie, I had to make a decision". He said, "I should have stopped but it wasn't finished, so I had to take a chance and complete it". He said, "I took my last decision, and ... it's mucked up". He gave me a certificate saying I couldn't work for six months, and after a few months I went back to him and he did another operation – a TURP. He cleared it through the prostate into the bladder so then I was able to return to work. Going through the prostate they take samples and it didn't show cancer.

Rising ... and falling PSA

A few years later my GP ordered a blood test including a PSA which showed 27 and I said, "What does that mean?" and he said, "Well, it means that your antibodies are fighting something – it could be cancer, it could be something else". He said, "If you get ... a, um ... if your bladder gets infected, it could make the PSA rise". He said there are many, many reasons but the thing we worry about is cancer and so I went back to the urologist who did a biopsy – without anaesthetic, without anything ... quite painful ... but he said, "Hang on there, old chappie, I'm just going to go through and grab a piece". "Bang ... snap ...", they knock you out now. So the eight samples showed no cancer, and then the PSA dropped. Because I was not so well informed about everything as now, I waited 18 months, it was out of my hands, and, I'm not ashamed to say that, because of the biopsy, and the pain, I thought, well, I want to avoid that. I was not told it was important to get more PSA tests or biopsies.

So then it rose to 38 and I had another biopsy which showed cancer and the Gleason reading – we thought he said seven, but later learned it was six. Our GP got a letter from the specialist saying, "Craig is not a candidate for the radiation, so I'm putting him on hormone treatment and I will inject him every six months and I'll get you to inject him the other three-month intervals between". So I did that for four years and I had awful side-effects with … and, um … well, I love working around the house and I could get bags of concrete – cement, and I couldn't get them out of the car; I had no strength.

"You've got 12 months to live!"

And, um … so how did I get off the hormones? … the PSA started to rise again, after my heart surgery so, OK, when you're in that treatment, you read 0.7, 0.9, and I attended a support group on the Sunshine Coast, until one was started at home. When the PSA started rising again, I saw a new urologist – oh, that's right, my specialist retired so I went to another leading urologist.

This urologist did not examine me or do any tests but declared I had had it and he said, "You've got 12 months to live!". We were not satisfied with his verdict so we saw another urologist who was in the hospital in Brisbane. About the same time a man working for the radiation from the Brisbane Hospital came to the Sunshine Coast and gave a talk at the Support Meeting. "Any questions?" Well, I didn't have any questions then but when he finished I gave him my background and he said, "Well you're a candidate for radiation". But I said, "I've got a letter at home …" but he said, "Well, it's changed so much now that the new doctors coming through have an entirely different mindset to the old doctors". … The Brisbane urologist said he couldn't see how the Sunshine Coast urologist came to the decision without any tests and he would restage me. He got in touch with the radiologist and recommended radiation for me. That was five years after I was first diagnosed and it's been five years since then.

Decision-making stress

I was diagnosed only by him looking at me. And I said, "How long have I got to live?" and he said, "You've only got 12 months". And I said, "What happens?" and he said, "Ring me and I'll give you narcotics to ease the pain." So he obviously wanted us to go because he had a full room, and then, I was delivering books next day to the various nursing homes around here, and I sat down, and – I'm in shock – said to the guy delivering the books with me, "You go ahead, Major, I'm resting here" and I sat down and thought, I'll ring a Brisbane urologist Dr MacDonald up because I saw him treating and speaking so kindly to the man in the bed next to me, I remembered that. When I came home Dianne, my wife, said … (I came home positive that I was going to get a second opinion) … so Dianne said, "I have been talking with a support group I read about in the paper and they said we should see someone else, so I phoned for an appointment with that nice urologist in Brisbane". And I said I was going to come home and say to ring! So we saw Dr MacDonald. In the meantime we went to the support group and you had to stand and give your story and I told them mine. Dr X's name came up and they booed, hissed and booed, and had all these stories of him, including the man who is living at the end of my street here. When he saw him, he told him he was going to die and he said, "How long have I got?", and he said, "Well, you're 79 – how long do you expect to live?" It was unbelievable. So I knew then I was sent to the wrong person. So I saw Dr MacDonald and he said, "I don't see how he can make a diagnosis on that scant evidence", so I told him about this radiologist speaking at our meeting. He gave him a ring so he said, um, "Yes, I'm referring him to you for radiation". So, and in the meantime … radiation had been pretty horrendous in the past; everyone had these stories of being totally beggared after radiation – massive burns – but now it has improved so much we feel that, by delaying the radiation for the few years, I got through reasonably unscathed even though I had bad side-effects for quite a few years. The PSA had dropped quite considerably before the radiation but we decided to go ahead with it anyway and it dropped further after it.

"I'm in the last lap"

Sometimes the pain is so much that I scream and cry and wish I'd die. I'll be lucky to be here in a few months' time. I'm starting this treatment Tuesday. Ah … well, I'm in dire straits. I'm in the last lap.

My growing spirituality

Dianne has always been a practising Christian, always going to church, went to church on her own, without her husband. She decided with me that she wasn't going to church without me. So I got the Bible out. It was very easy to find in the Bible something to laugh at, criticise, like Abraham and Sarah, like, hundreds of examples you can poke fun at ... I'm probably not as bad as I'm making out, but I did say that the Bible, you couldn't live like that because, um, the angry God, and then we, ah ... I could see how much she missed the church so we started going to church and then, um, I probably, um, I probably turned around about 10 years ago.

I was looking at the Bible – reading it, generally without a thought to criticise but to find some truth. Everyone our age knows of Helen Keller. We heard a sermon and Helen Keller was mentioned, and so we got the book we knew she had written about her religion called now *A light to my darkness* but was originally *My Religion*. Anyway, we read the book and could see something special there. I loved it and read it and re-read it so my wife bought me a copy. Her first marriage was in what they call the New Church. This was formed by a society of people who read Emanuel Swedenborg's writings. He actually wrote 32 books – about a thousand-odd pages in each book – mostly on the Old Testament. So, I worked it out as 30 words for every word in the Old Testament. He really has explained how to understand the Old Testament and the Gospels and Revelation. He never tried to preach or start anything. He just wrote for people to read or not read.

You just couldn't help but get involved with Helen Keller. About this time I had discovered that my ancestor, James McKnight, was a great theologian and had done a new translation of all the Epistles. These rare books in a set of six volumes were available through the internet and they also had his biography in the first volume. We purchased these and I was inspired by reading his commentaries knowing that he was a direct great-great-great-grandfather so I felt a connection. So it was Divine Providence that my family history came to light about the same time I was searching. I'm thinking that a miracle's happened, and I think it's a miracle from heaven, from above. Previously I had not even heard of him. My spirituality commenced slowly but for Dianne it was reignited.

I'm just thinking that this had been pre-arranged that Helen Keller would be introduced to the writings of Emmanuel Swedenborg when a dear friend translated them into Braille for her. So I thought this man's special. So we were able to get many, many books – more modern translations of Swedenborg as he wrote 200 years ago and in Latin. The more I read, the more it appeared that, that … I haven't embraced the New Church, I've met many people from the New Church and I find them all to be inspirational type of people.

I wanted to find out more but I found it very difficult to find out more because I was 75 at the time, roughly, and my brain's not as nearly good as it was – my brain's probably never any good – and Emanuel Swedenborg is not easy to read, so I found it very difficult to pick up one of his books and to read it and immediately get inspired, because he is a fact man; now that's probably putting it wrongly … in essence, the main thing was that it took away my fear of death. He wrote a book – *Heaven and Hell* – about him visiting heaven. I must say I haven't read the whole lot, I've read bits and pieces; Dianne's probably read it two or three times. I've got to be honest, I'm not really sure he did visit heaven but certain he had some sort of experience or vision.

Spirituality in practice

I think I am a reasonably pleasant person to live with. I still become unpleasant at odd times … but this has helped me have a greater communion with God. Before, I never had a clue about God; I never had a clue about Jesus …

I think church itself is … you know, you get some wonderful sermons, you get other sermons; sometimes it's a pain in the neck to get ready to go. There's the social side of church, there's the wonderful people you meet in church, but generally … generally the sermons really don't lift me up, no.

What does lift me up is being able to talk things over with Dianne; she's very matter-of-fact, and can get me back on the right leg, the right road, by a few simple words. And also today I had 51 minutes of talking with the Support Group Convenor. He's the Reverend John Tills. He's a prostate sufferer. He is one of the most down-to-earth Christians Dianne and I have ever met. He's to the point. He makes being a Christian so simple. He says, "Love the Lord and love your neighbour". He says, "What's hard about that?" And he's helped some homosexuals who were moving house and he does a weekly service, but some people criticised him for helping them, and he said, "I'm here to help people"; he said, "Someone else judges them".

"Things like that lift you up"

My spiritualty has never decreased. I wish it would increase. I think that, unless I can reignite it, I think at the minute I'm stagnant. I struggle intellectually. I'm not capable of getting up high. I wish I could. There are dozens and dozens of really great books I wish I could just pick them up and spend four hours reading them but I can't. I find that after 15 minutes my mind wavers and I read things in there that really inspire me. I feel disappointed about this. I really think I should have started years before when I was in the wilderness. Yeah, disappointed.

I wish my spirituality would become more intense. I know I keep bringing up my partner, my wife, all the time. She's very, very spiritual compared with me. Very spiritual. I'd love to lift myself closer to her. OK. I got lifted up yesterday by the dentist, the x-ray people, the lady who took us into the place where I'm having this treatment next Tuesday. I got lifted up by Reverend Tills yesterday when I mentioned spirituality. We had a lady come in next door and she sat there and you could see kindness all round her. Things like that lift you up.

The only greater support I would like comes from my soul. With better knowledge. I think it is up to me to lift, not other people. But Dianne is my crutch.

When the chips were down

There were times when the chips were down and the back was against the wall; you really wanted to get the books out and read and get help, but I notice in the last four or five months I'm not doing it like I used to. I notice that my memory is really getting, ah … I also like watching and listening to (religious) CDs, DVDs and sermons. I have a lot of wonderful friends who call in often. I love the company and chatting about things and reminiscing about the boxing in Australia and past champions. Ex-boxers are a fine group of people. I follow the racing on Saturdays and my interest in horses goes back to my school days. Happy memories of caravan trips with my wife are important as we made the last trip late 2009 and we knew it would be our last and have recently sold our van.

Wayne

Wayne lived by himself in a retirement village. For a man of 85, he was exceptionally active in the village and in his church. He was articulate and focussed.

First signs

I, for some years, had a problem with an unexplained pain on the left side of my penis, and I was fortunate that on one occasion when I went to see my GP, in whom I had a great deal of faith, that he wasn't available and I saw one of the doctors that was standing in for him. He said straight away that at your age, which would have been somewhere in the mid-50s at the time, he said that I should have a PSA around 5, and, of course, it happened to be somewhere near 8, 9. It was elevated. So he said, "Well, we won't worry about it at this stage but we'll keep an eye on it" and it continued to rise. When it got up to 14, I was sent for a biopsy of the prostate, and, I'll say with hindsight, unfortunately for me, that in those days they carried out a four-needle biopsy which only covered 80% of the gland and my first biopsy was clear. It was found necessary to have a second biopsy done in six months. The second biopsy showed that the prostate cancer was certainly there, and not only was it there but it was already outside of the gland. I was unfortunate that I couldn't have the gland removed and be cured. I was put on a course of the drug Androcur to see how the cancer would respond to that. After six weeks it was found that the PSA had dropped to 1.2. Oh, and I thought that was a magic figure and I thought this was something I was going to be on for the rest of my life until the urologist hit me straight between the eyes. He said, "Now that we've proved that, we've got to remove the source of the hormones – the source of the hormones being your testicles". And I said, "Well, what if I don't have the operation?" "Well", he said, "it's the rest of your life we're talking about."

"The whole ground was taken away"

Well, the whole ground was taken away out from under my feet. But, at the same time, I couldn't do anything else but stare the reality of it in the face if I was going to live for any reasonable length of time from that point on. I had to have the operation. So I just said, "When do we have the operation?" By this time, I might add, my wife had developed Alzheimer's disease and she wasn't available to discuss anything with me and, unfortunately, I had to make all these decisions on my own and this made things much more difficult as far as I was concerned because a problem shared is a problem at least halved, isn't it? Anyway I went ahead and had the operation in a reasonably short time. I would have been about 70 at the time, I suppose. I went through everything they tell you that you go through – hot flushes (the Americans call them "flashes"). They are not very pleasant, but …

Comfort of the church

I had come back to my church some time prior to this and I was very, very grateful that I had because it was the source of not simply comfort, but enormous support because a) I had a priest to talk to, and b) the Lord was there to help – every moment of every day and I found I could get over all these problems given they were as difficult as they were, especially the hot flushes. They can happen at any time. They just weren't pleasant.

By talking to the priest at least I was sharing my problems with someone, and then by praying you get the comfort. The Lord's hand is comfort. It is available to you at all times to give comfort. It is real. It is not pie in the sky. It is real and you take the comfort from your prayers. You can lift your head up and say, right, the Lord's with me. I'm going to cope with this with His help. I was able to cope.

"I was no longer any use to them whatsoever!"

When I look back over the whole time, nothing was done as far as treatment was concerned. I wasn't offered any treatment; they simply said that we go ahead and see what develops and nothing developed virtually over the whole time. I might say that the PSA, after the removal of the testicles, went down to 0.1 and remained at 0.1 over a period of some years – quite some years. But at the back of my mind I always knew that the day was going to come that this was going to lift off the bottom, that I had not had a cure; it was just on hold. I had a PSA every six months and finally it went to 0.2, 0.5, then 1.0 and slowly progressed upwards from there.

It came to the point where the urologist was on a panel of doctors who were looking for men with a rising PSA and they wanted to test a new drug called Denosumab to prevent the spread of the cancer to the bones. They asked me if I would go on to that and I said, "Certainly I will". I went on to that program, visiting a Russian lady doctor at the hospital every month for nearly three years. Everything seemed to go along very well. I had bone scans, MRIs and this was a very good thing as far as I was concerned because they had a close look at my progress which I wouldn't have got if I had not been on the program. But the day came when one of the bone scans indicated that I had a secondary in one of my pelvic bones. I was no longer any use to them whatsoever for their program.

More disappointment

I was thoroughly disappointed. I had developed a very nice relationship with this lady doctor. She was comforting – someone to go to every month to have someone to talk to. I knew that that had come to an end. So it was most unfortunate as far as I was concerned.

However, I was still going to the doctor who was overseeing my whole program; he was still my urologist. I was still going to see him every six months anyway. I think it took probably over 12 months and he said to me that there was a panel of doctors – of which he was one – from different disciplines that were looking at what he called difficult cases. He said he would like to refer my file to that panel to see what came up in discussions from different points of view. Then as recently as September last year (2010) I had a letter from that panel saying that there was a novel treatment being looked at by a group of doctors in California based on your own immune system and they intended to develop a vaccine and that they would probably offer me this novel treatment. Well, that was the last I heard of that until recently when I asked about it and they said that, as with some new things, funding dries up and that seems to be what has happened.

I had a back pain – this is quite recent, going back only three or four weeks ago – and I intended to see my physio who had treated the same area of my back three or four months back successfully. My GP said, "No, I want a bone scan done before you do that". (I hadn't had a bone scan done for about two years.) They found many more secondaries, in my ribs this time and virtually the whole length of my spine. He said no more physio; bones could be broken. That's the point that I'm virtually at now.

Treatments – "We'll see what happens"

I have seen my urologist again and he has given me a new drug which is to help, in his own words, in knocking down the secondaries and bringing the PSA down. I'm sorry, there was a point in July of last year where they had suggested that 10 days of radiation might be useful; and it was. My PSA dropped from 52 down to 14 by the radiation. But one month later it was up to 16, another month it was up to 25. I asked my GP to lay it on the line – what's the score from here on? "Well", he said, "PSA is the story. If the PSA continues to go up at the same rate, you might have another 12 months to live, but if it levels out you might have another five years." When I told my urologist about that, he said, "Well, it's a brave doctor who will start talking about exact times". He said, "You might say six months but your patient's bouncing around still in two years' time." He said, "Sure, your PSA's increasing which is not a good thing" (this was about the time of the new drug) "so we'll see what happens with that".

Spiritual activity and slow physical decline

Getting back to spirituality … I was very blessed in that, quite close to the time when I was first diagnosed, I lived here at a retirement village and we had a church service once a week in the middle of the week. They needed an assistant, and in Anglican terms they wanted a liturgical assistant (LA), to assist at the altar. I was asked, even though I was 70 years of age, would I take on that role. Well, I thought, I'd never done this before in my life but it was something certainly I would very much like to do, and I did. The Lord has blessed me greatly because every week I'm involved in a minimum of two services here and at St Alban's on Thursdays and then I take my turn in our own church which is at least once a month. Sometimes I sit in for other people when they are not able to be there, so I'm able to be part of the sanctuary party for the service, which is a lot better than simply sitting in the pew.

I think, myself, that I've been slowly declining as far as my physical strength is concerned – my legs and my back – and had I not been participating as an LA, I think I would have just given up maybe two years ago, but I've got the strength through my faith and from the Lord; He can hold you up.

I did my LA work here today at the retirement village and, even though I'm knocked out because I have to do a patrol around the wings for people who are bed-bound, and that's physically exhausting, but I'm still able to do it. I have to rest most Wednesday and Thursday afternoons, but nevertheless I'm still able to do it and, with the Lord's help, I'll continue to do it for at least some little time to come.

Spiritual strength

I think my religious activities only strengthen me. Just as an example, I belong to a group of people who meet on a Monday night fortnightly for prayer and praise. For a time, the host and hostess of that group had health problems and I just said, "Well, my little unit doesn't hold very many people but you're welcome to come to my place if you want to". There were only three of us here on Monday night this week, but each one gets something out of coming. I certainly do. I would not like to see the early demise of that group.

My spirituality has been increasing and the closer I get to the point where I know my lifespan is getting shorter and shorter ... oh, I'm welcoming that fact because of what I have taken from my Christianity. I welcome the time when I can meet my Lord.

Wayne's worship

I've got formal worship in church each Sunday and I've got formal worship here every Wednesday morning, and Thursday mornings over at St Alban's. Apart from that, there are times throughout each day when you see something. You'll be outside and you might see a bird fly over, or you might see a particular formation of clouds. It just strikes you that you thank the Lord for the beauty He has created. Those things come to mind. Then, apart from that, I have a time each night before I go to sleep; I've got three different daily devotionals – although I don't use them all each night. There's a Scripture reading and then a discussion on that Scripture reading by the author. One of them is Martin Luther. I enjoy his point of view coming down through the centuries. And then there are always Bible readings. We have a church lectionary and I always do the daily readings. There's a Psalm for the day before I go to sleep each night. There was a time when I tried to do a morning prayer before breakfast but I just found that the world sort of rushes in every morning when you wake up – there are so many things to do and I wasn't able to keep that up. I've never got into meditation; it's something that would be worthwhile to do.

Spiritual beginnings

I'll go right back to my childhood for a start. My parents were not church-goers. But my mother saw to it, not so much for my two older brothers but for my sister who is three years older than me (and I am the youngest) but my sister and I, wherever we lived – and we had moved three or four times – my mother saw to it that my sister and I went to the nearest Sunday School and it didn't matter what denomination it was. When, later in my life, when I had time to sort these things out for myself, I was so thankful that I had that Sunday School background. Even when I was in the army I always looked for church parade. I even got myself into trouble one time when I insisted on going to church parade. The thread was always there because of that early training in Sunday School even though I drifted away from the church partly because my wife developed agoraphobia early in our marriage. Actually, she was a church-goer when I met her and I started going to the Anglican Church because she was Anglican. I had not been going to an Anglican Church at that time, and I was so thankful because I love the Anglican ritual and I love the structure of the Anglican service.

Coping with the stress of prostate cancer

My faith – it's always there. It's not something I think about. I think it's there in the background all the time and when there are these stress points and, certainly, I'll put it this way: it's happened three or four times now and in one of them I had a complete blockage and I had to have an emergency operation, and what you go through prior to this emergency operation I was praying. That's helped me many times when I've been waiting for things such as operations (and I've been through a number of them over the years): prayer prior to an operation has been a priority as far as I am concerned.

Some activities – lifting the spirit, or just hobbies?

I wonder if you would call some activities spiritualities or whether you would tend to call them interests. I've had an interest as an amateur astronomer and I've had an interest as an amateur wireless operator. Those two things can absorb you completely and you can switch off from the world.

They used to lift me. Not so much being a ham, partly because of the sunspot situation. Old spotty face up there hasn't got a spotty face at the present time. Our radio waves go straight through; they don't come back. As far as astronomy is concerned, it does because it's the most absorbing thing outside anything else I've ever done. It lifts you up and takes you away from any problem you might have.

Continued spiritual support

I've been very fortunate that the priest of our parish who asked me to become a liturgical assistant, I had quite a close relationship with him but I've had an even closer relationship with the two priests that have followed him in the parish and especially the one we've got at the present time. I've got all the spiritual support that I could possibly hope for from our current priest. He's a wonderful fella.

All in all, I feel quite blessed in that my illness has curtailed what might otherwise have been a more active self-seeking life. The necessity of being at the nursing home daily during my wife's long illness gave me the opportunity to develop my own long association as a volunteer with the occupational therapy staff and dealing with other people's problems diverts you from your own.

Colin

Colin was very welcoming. He was excited to tell his story because he believed he had something to contribute. He lived with his wife and two small, sometimes noisy dogs in a very comfortable home. He was a well-organised person and this showed in the way his story was constructed. He was 79 at the time of the interview.

The beginning of the journey

I had very little spirituality. I left school and then I had 40 years of nothing. And then I developed spirituality from then on so it was a big gap. I had no background of Christ or the Bible or anything, really. When I left school it was put out of my mind so I had that long gap. So when I come into it now it's all new.

Probably about six years ago the doctor did a complete blood test and the PSA showed up there. So that was the start of it; so then he got me into a urologist and he had a look at it and did all the tests on me. The Gleason score was seven and the PSA was 39 which they said was pretty high. So we did some more tests where they found that the cancer had metastasised to the bone. So I've got a spot on the sacroiliac joint which is where it is now and it hasn't changed.

Going back to the urologist, he gave me a book to read on all the different treatments for prostate cancer, and the alternatives. I read through it pretty carefully. I like to know what they are going to do to me. There was one there that looked fairly good to me; it wasn't invasive. It meant getting an injection every three months. It was the hormone therapy treatment. So I went through the book and marked it all out and highlighted this particular one. When I went back to him, he looked at me and said, "Well, we've got a few options. In your case it has escaped the capsule from the prostrate and it's into the bone. We can do chemotherapy or radiation". I looked at him and he said, "Hmm. There's one other one and that's hormone therapy treatment". And I said, "What chances have I got with it?" and he said, "Very good". So I opened the book and showed it to him – this was the one I had already highlighted. So I said, "We'll go for that". So we started on the injections and every three months I go around to get one. The PSA has dropped back to 0.2 and for the last six years it's been pretty close to 0.4 or 0.5. So it's running at that and, while it's maintained at that, we'll stick with it. I've had about 25 injections – which is six years. He's quite rapt in it. He said I must be one of the lucky ones. I said, "Well, I have a lot of help". That's where I am now and that's where it all came about.

Force in spirituality

I wasn't a Christian at that time; I was a hypnotist practising in sports. I used to work on sportspeople and that type of thing and there was one guy I used to watch on TV. His name was Benny Hinn. He was an American evangelist. I used to call Pamela, my wife, out and say, "Have a look at this; he's unbelievable at what he does". I used to watch him because I wanted to learn how he did it. I thought he was the best hypnotist I'd ever seen. This went on for a while and, in that time Pamela became a Christian, got baptised and did all the things. I wasn't quite ready for it at that stage. My uncle was living in Sydney and he was getting a bit old so I thought I'll go down and see him. At the same time Benny Hinn was having a crusade in Sydney and that was 2006. I booked in and went down and went to the crusade. I got in there and there must have been 1,000 people there. I got a seat that was looking right over the stage and the music came on and everybody started to sing and dance and wave their arms and carry on and I thought, what am I doin' here? It was quite amazing and Benny Hinn walked out on the stage and I look around and think, hey, I'm doin' the same thing. They'd got me. There was a lot of power there and a lot of force. I know that was the first time I felt the Holy Spirit. So that's where the spirituality started. When I came back from there I was convinced that, OK Benny, you must be getting a lot of help from above, from the Lord, and I thought, wow, this is pretty amazing stuff. The people Pamela was doing the Bible study with, they talked to me about joining and I said, no, I'm not quite ready; I need to do a couple of things.

I didn't tell Pamela. I had to read the Bible and I had to get baptised, then I'd do the rest of it. So that's my journey in that area. We found a church.

Pamela did the churches. She went to about four churches. She didn't like them all that much so she decided to go to one out at Jindalee. When she got out there she came home, she said, "Wow, that's really good; it's just like being at home". So we went out there and joined in with everything. We went to Bible study at Church and in home groups and it was really good. And then I discovered that, OK, something happened when I was in Sydney – whatever it was, whether it was a very good doctor or I was getting a lot of help – and my PSA hasn't changed in four years.

No prostate symptoms

I have no trouble with the waterworks – it's all working fine and I've got no symptoms. I had to go and ask the doctor how I should feel. I feel very good. I've lost a fair bit of weight but looking at the hormone therapy treatment and what it does to you, you lose your muscle mass and bone mass as the side-effects and I kept talking to him about that and asking what's the treatment. Finally he put me on to Actonel which is Calcium and Vitamin B combined tablets, so I keep those up. I didn't like losing weight. I lost about 10 kilos. But I still do the gardens and lawns; I still do weights four days a week and this seems to keep me fairly active. At the moment, all of the treatment is through hormone therapy.

A positive approach

Well, I have it cancer and the first thing I thought of was how can I beat it? I'm pretty positive with what I do and I said, well, what's the options?, let's look at them and see where we can go and what we can do. So I looked at everything that was available to me and that's how I decided I would treat it. I wasn't a Christian at that stage.

I had a bone density x-ray. That's just a while ago. I wasn't impressed with that either. They did the left side and I have the problem on the right side. They said everything is all right. They were quite happy with what they were doing. I might not be happy but I think they should know what they're doing.

Prostate cancer and my spirituality

There is probably a direct relationship between my cancer and spirituality. I pray for a miracle and a healing, and I know that my inner self is a lot stronger. I have no fears or doubts. I'm here now and everything's been done that I could possibly do and I'm in the Lord's hands. I'm quite confident in what's happened.

The Bible is the greatest source of my spirituality. Most of the passages in the Bible are related to "ask and ye shall receive"; "the Lord gives"; "the Lord is a healing God". He is very caring so I know I'm in good hands.

Benny Hinn is someone who gives me a tremendous amount of encouragement. I like his teachings, I like his manner and I know he does a lot of good. He's one of the top evangelists in America. He does crusades throughout the world every month. He doesn't say, "You've got to do this or you've got to do that". He's got a good manner about him. If they start to tell me what I've got to do, or don't do, I kind of back off. He gives me what I need – put it that way.

We go to church on Sundays. It's a very good service. We've got a very good preacher. He's a teacher and a preacher. The people there are very good people. We're very comfortable there. It's like being at a family reunion.

Spiritual growth

My spirituality has increased because I had nothing until I started four years ago. We did look at a couple of things when we came up here from Melbourne. We settled into the house and everything and we got involved in sports and all that type of stuff and as I got a bit older the sports faded out a bit. We both knew there was something better. We were looking for something; we didn't know what it was. We looked at Buddhist and Tai Chi and a couple of other ones, you know, but nothing was there that we needed or wanted. Then we met a lady who used to walk past here every morning. We had a blow-out with a water pipe and she knocked on the door and told us we had water everywhere. Then we got talking. She was a Christian and Pamela got involved with her and they went to home Bible study which was very good and I got the backwash of this all the time which was pretty good, and it developed from there. That's how Pamela got baptised and became a Christian. Then when I got baptised and became a Christian and Pamela found the church she liked, I said, "That's good enough for me".

The cancer has been on hold for six years. My spirituality has helped me a lot because it has given me a good mindset. I've got no doubts. I've done everything in my power, and the Lord's help, to keep it there, to lie dormant. I expect it to go away. I asked the doctor after getting the PSA report and he reads it and says, "That's good", and I said, "Well I expected it to go away, to be zero". He looked at me as if I'm a bit strange. I honestly expect it to be zero one day.

I've never really felt down during the time of my cancer. I would say I get a little doubtful when I go for the blood tests. It's there at the end of the three-month period and I feel, ah … let it be nothing. I don't do anything special before my tests. I know I'm going, what is going to happen and I'll get the report off the doctor. I expect him to tell me that it's gone down. I have a good mindset with it before my tests. I know where I'm goin' and I know what I'm doin'. I know it's there; it hasn't gone away. But it's not going to get me!

Practising spirituality

I tell you what, it's, … I'm in a sports club. I compete every weekend – Saturday – with a group of guys there. Their manner and attitude has changed around me. They used to come out with all the dirty, filthy jokes, and now they don't tell them. I'm quite amazed at that really, because one of the guys has a joke every week, every day, you know, and he said to me last Saturday, "Oh, Colin, I've got a good joke for you – it's all right, it's a Christian joke". The people around me have changed. It's quite amusing really. I think this change in others has happened because of the change within me, the change within my manner, aura, whatever you like to call it. I can't think of the word. Something has changed around me because my whole life has changed. For about 40 years I worked in pubs; my life was in pubs so you know what I dealt with. I dealt with different things then so my life has really changed and the people around me have changed. It's a good feeling.

Physical and spiritual support

I went to the prostate cancer meeting every month and they have some good lectures there and some good people and people give testimonials about what they are doing but there wasn't enough input. Everyone wanted to talk about their own problems, not solving the problems and moving forward into another area where they'd come up with treatments or herbs or new work, or something like that. I felt they just weren't going in the direction I wanted to go. But I listened and learnt everything I could but I just dropped out of it. But I still get the cancer magazine which is very good. If you read it there's so much information in it. It's way above me in technical terms but I can read what progress they're making, what new things are coming out, where they're going – but it's all key news of the future. I still like to read it. I enjoy reading about the stuff they're doing now – the vaccine they've perfected and are still testing. OK, the thing works, it's wonderful, it's wow, wow, wow, but 10 years down the track we might get it.

Spirituality during stress

Probably the stress points have been every three months when I get the needle. I know I'm going to get that, but I can switch off it, I can cut it out. I use my hypnosis. I know I'm going to get it. I can deaden the side. I don't feel it. I go and get it and I'm out in 10 minutes. Sometimes he talks, sometimes he doesn't.

My hypnosis began with sport – I was involved in sports for 50 years. Concentration and focussing are two of the main things. We used to get psychologists coming in to give us a lecture on something. They were never related to what we were doing. Then, when I gave up work, I got involved as a coach – level 3. I ran into a guy who was involved with hypnosis and I said, "Do you think I can do it?" and he said, "Yes, you would have no trouble doing it". I think there was about 300 hours of practical, hands-on hypnosis. I learnt a lot from it and then developed my own techniques and methods which I started to pursue and I've used it right through. It gave me a lot of insight into people and a lot of control over my own body – switching off, pain, deadening areas, all that type of stuff. Pretty open really. It's a wonderful media to use in a lot of places.

Hypnosis is probably part of my spirituality, because it is a relationship between you and a person. They've got to have faith in you before you can do it. They give themselves to you; they put themselves in your hands. And I have done a little bit of healing. The hypnosis and the healing come in together, and spirituality. If you say it's in God's name you're healed, or, if the healing process is in your mind, it is accelerated. You can feel the power – the mind taking over ruling the body. Probably where I am, I've got to be a little bit careful in what I do. I'm not stepping forward and doing it; I'm there. I can do things with people that are very good but I'm not going to get up on the stage and do it. There's a lady praying over a girl. I was there in the group and they said to do something so I put both hands on her knee and I said, "Feel the power of healing". When she was finished she was outside rubbing her leg and I said, "How are you going?" and she said, "Oh, really good. The leg's still hot". So something worked. She said that it feels good; it was very hot.

My spiritual source

I only have one source of spirituality. I think there is only one God – three people. We have the Father, the Son and the Holy Spirit. The main source is the Holy Spirit and He's the one that guides you and helps you. I'm only new at this but I listen to Benny Hinn. He was on this morning. He was talking about the spirit and soul. There's the Holy Spirit, my spirit, my soul and my body. It's quite interesting really how he broke it up, how one intercedes with the other.

I think my spirituality is a gift. It is a gift. My hypnosis, healing and spirituality are all part of the one.

Ben

Ben lived by himself in an apartment near the coast. He was anxious to tell his story because so much of his life, especially around his prostate cancer journey, was disturbing for him.

No symptoms

I didn't have any symptoms at all. There had been bits in the news about prostate cancer and I'd never been tested and someone told me I should go along to my doctor, my GP, and ask him to be tested so I did that. He'd never suggested prior to that that I have a test. Twelve months prior to this I was feeling really tired at work and went to my GP and told him that. He put me on a course of vitamin tablets. I was also a bit low on iron so I took some iron tablets for a while. Initially it helped me and I got over that tiredness but twelve months later someone told me I should go and have the tests so I had a test for bowel cancer and a few other tests but I never had the prostate cancer test so I went along and said to him, "Can I have this test?" So he did the digital examination first, then I had the blood test, then it came back and I had a PSA of 26 which he said was pretty high because the average is about 2 or 3, I think. I was astounded, and then I had a scan and it confirmed that I was just full of cancer.

It was in August 2009 when I went to my GP and he said I needed to see a specialist straight away and it was the next day. Normally it takes three months to get in to a specialist but, because it was so bad, they took me the following day. I had more scans and the results came back and confirmed that the cancer was really bad.

"Just blurt it out!"

They took samples and they discovered I had the aggressive cancer and they were able to confirm that the cancer had already spread to the vas deferens and the lymph nodes. When my specialist saw the x-rays, he turned to me – well, he wasn't saying anything and I said to him, "You're not saying anything" and I said, "What's wrong?", and he said, "I don't know how to tell you" and I said, "Well, just blurt it out!" and he said,

"Well, I don't think you can be cured". And, of course, that came as a hell of a shock to me from having no symptoms to all of a sudden having a death sentence. And then he said, "We're going to have to remove the prostate. It's going to be a huge operation. You need to get yourself as fit as you possibly can". But I was already fit because I was working at the time and doing a lot of walking during the day and was really fit anyway.

I was just due to have holidays and I asked if I had to be operated on now and should I wait and they said, "No, go and have your holiday and when you come back we'll have the operation".

A state of shock

So I was in a state of shock. So I rang my son. I had a son living in Bendigo, Victoria, and I thought, how am I going to get through this?; how am I going to get through this operation? So, I went on sick leave from work straight away because I had to have this operation and I needed a recovery time afterwards. About 10 days before I had the operation I decided to go and see my mother in New Zealand for four days. Then I went to visit my son and that gave me the strength to help me get through the operation because it was going to be a huge operation and I just had to find the strength to be able to get through and that enabled me to have the strength to survive the operation. So I had my holiday and came back and had the operation. I had the prostate removed.

I was in private health, in the Mercy Private Hospital. I was there for four nights, then allowed to go home. I had a catheter for two weeks. I had to stay with an elderly male friend that I knew who was good enough to let me stay at his place for a couple of weeks after the operation. I was able to survive the operation – wearing a catheter I didn't like; it was horrible, actually – I was so pleased to get rid of that. After that I remained on sick leave because it takes months to get over an operation like that. You have difficulties with walking to begin with. There was also incontinence that went on for about three months – that's not very pleasant. You have to do exercises to try to help strengthen the pelvic floor. Eventually, over time, I regained my strength.

Treatments and tests

I also decided to go to a Chinese herbalist. For six weeks I had a course of Chinese herbs which I used to boil up every day and drink the mixture. That really gave me a boost. The herbalist also gave me some Ginseng. I boiled water and put the dried Ginseng into a mug and drank that. That really lifted my spirit and it was of real benefit to me. I got all my energy back and I started to feel good. This was for six months after the operation.

After the operation I was having blood tests to see what level the PSA was. About six weeks after the operation the level had gone down to almost zero. Every six weeks I had more blood tests.

At the end of April it showed that the cancer was spreading at an alarming rate; that it was actually doubling every six weeks. So the day I got these results, he said, "I'll start you on hormone injections straight away". I had to take hormone tablets for a few weeks and then I had to have an injection every three months. To begin with it kept the level right down – almost undetectable. I had a blood test on Monday of last week and I got the results back yesterday. I am now back to square one. I'm at the same level today as I was almost 10 months ago. The hormone treatment has started to become ineffective in the sense that the cancer is starting to take over again. It's now 0.19. The previous reading was 0.05 so it's doubled and almost doubled again.

So I had an injection yesterday. The specialist said, "You'll possibly have one more injection", then said, "I'd like you to think about having some chemo". I said I wasn't very interested in that. Prior to having hormone treatment they suggested I have radiotherapy. They said there was only a 5% chance that this would cure me and that there was a 20% risk that it would damage some other organs. I was not prepared to take that risk. I wouldn't feel comfortable if I damaged my bowel and if had to have a colostomy bag. I talked it over with my son and he said, "Don't put yourself through that". So that's when I decided to go for the hormone treatment. But now the specialist is talking about the chemo and I'm reluctant to do that because I was diagnosed with terminal right from the start and there was little chance of me being cured.

A tough journey

I was in the situation where I live by myself; I had my son and I had close friends but I found it very difficult, so I actually turned to God – I'm not a religious person – but I turned to God to give me strength. I prayed every night and every morning in the hope that I could be cured. For a long time I'd be feeling really well but over the last month I have not been feeling all that well. I wake up during the night and I feel ill, sick in the stomach. Some mornings I feel light-headed and I can't walk in a straight line. To be honest with you, I've actually stopped praying now. I can't explain why because it was just something that … like I said, I wasn't a religious person but I turned to that in the hope that, yes, you haven't got much when you're diagnosed with a terminal illness. It hits you like a rock; there's not much to grasp hold of, really. So that's why I started praying.

And another way I was able to cope with it was to tell as many people as I knew or even some people I didn't know all that well that I had this cancer, as I found it was too big a burden for me to carry and that lightened the load. Well, in a funny sort of way I wanted to spread it around, although I didn't want to spread the illness, but I wanted to spread the story, I suppose, just to take the weight off my shoulders because when you are diagnosed with a terminal illness it's just a huge burden and, yes, it's really hard to cope with. We all cope with it differently. Yes, that was my way of coping with it, yes … it's, ah …it's shattering, especially at my age.

"It's hard to accept"

I feel that my GP really let me down. He was a professional and he should have known. There's a lot of people do know, but there's a lot of people don't know, like myself, that there's a lot of people saying that even at 40 men should be tested every 12 months, and, yes, I felt very let down by the doctor because he never ever said. But then I went up and saw another specialist in Brisbane and I mentioned that to him and he said, no, there's heaps of doctors who, if they saw a 56-year-old man walking in looking fit, they wouldn't even mention it. This is why I want to tell my story and maybe I can help someone else, because it's … just so … tragic. Like, my father lived to be 86, and, like, I'm thinking that maybe I'll reach that age, or maybe 90 and I've got another 30 years ahead of me; then, all of a sudden, I find that I'll be lucky to reach my 60th now. I feel robbed, really.

But I never really got angry about it; there's no point in doing that; you can carry on as much as you like but I just, I just had to come to terms with it. It's hard to accept but, you know, but that's the way it is and I've just got to cope with it as best I can.

I have had the support of a few close friends – a half a dozen or so. I also decided that when I was diagnosed with it I no longer worked so I've officially retired now. That's my decision – I just thought, you know, if I haven't got all that long to live, well, I'll just enjoy what little time I have left and make the most of it. I know of another case – he hasn't got prostate, he's got bowel cancer. He had an operation and is still choosing to work. That's his choice. I had an open prostatectomy. It was a about a 7-inch cut.

The lifts
I did have a lady friend who was very supportive. I was in a relationship with her prior to this. She helped me a lot. Every time I saw her it gave me strength. And then, of course, from one or two other friends, the guy that I met through my work as a delivery driver, he was very supportive. And my son. Not so much now but from the time I was diagnosed he was ringing every two or three days to see how I was. That gave me tremendous strength to cope with it.

Now it's not easy. There are times when I … I've been on antidepressants ever since I've been diagnosed with it and I'm still on antidepressants. And since I've been on hormones I've been on blood pressure pills – my blood pressure went right up. I guess I'll be on them for the rest of my life. I'll continue on the antidepressants because I wouldn't be able to cope at all otherwise. They have really been beneficial.

Support and counselling
I had one session with a support counsellor. I was offered six sessions actually. The counsellor was actually a woman. We talked for about 50 minutes. I just came away really angry. I think that, at the time, it was just focussing on my illness for that length of time. I didn't have any more after that. Recently I've had more stress because my mother is in a rest home in New Zealand. She has dementia and is not going to live much longer and

over the last month I've been pretty stressed out about that. The new GP that I have suggested that I have some general counselling with another organisation and I've found that very beneficial; it's really helped me. I did ring a prostate cancer support group when I was diagnosed and spoke to a gentleman there but I haven't gone down that path. I suppose if I had a partner I might have gone along and it might have been beneficial for my partner but sometimes I just like to keep to myself and maybe that's not the best way to go.

Painful side-effects

I've had a bit of sweating. Only today actually I'm all flushed in the face which I haven't had before, and also I can hardly walk today. I have aching legs and I've never had that before. When I first started I was sick in the stomach. I was really sick for three or four weeks. I took pain-killers to help me with this.

A need for strength

Often I really think about it and wonder how I'm going to gain the strength to get through this. Sometimes it might get all too much and then I might see friends and sometimes I might talk to them about it and they don't mind. A problem shared is a problem halved. It just works that way. When I was first diagnosed and told people, a number of people said to me, "I don't know what to say". And I said to them, "You don't have to say anything; I just have to get it off my chest". Some people were embarrassed, obviously. I said, "Don't worry about it". I just have to say it. It's helping me by saying it.

I bought a bike a month after the operation and now I try to ride my bike every day for exercise. I try to catch up with my friends and have a coffee; sometimes go out to breakfast – every Sunday actually with a group of about six of us.

A lot of times I keep to myself. Sometimes I have to push myself to get out. I don't know whether it's because of my star signs – I'm a Cancerian, I was born in June. Yes, I like to be by myself sometimes. Sometimes I'm just happy in my own environment; that's my way of coping with it. Sometimes I don't want to talk about it; other times I do tell people about it but I don't really want to burden other people with it. I can go to a counsellor and just blurt out whatever I like; it can bring tears to your eye but it doesn't really matter. Next day I've woken up feeling much better after getting that off my chest. It's not something I can burden my friends with but I can burden a counsellor with it. It's been very helpful, that. My GP says that I have so much on my plate with my mother, my cancer and that, I need to see a counsellor from time to time.

My mother and my son both gave me great inspiration. It's very difficult with my mother because when I told her I was sick she couldn't comprehend because she has dementia. She didn't know how bad it was for me. Now she doesn't really know how tragic it is. Even so, she gave me inspiration. She turned 90 in November 2010 and when I went over there we actually went out to lunch with our cousins. She was reasonably good but since then she has deteriorated a lot.

"I got the short straw!"
I just can't believe what's happening to her and to myself ... In some cases some people on hormone go for 10 years and still going. Studies have shown that 99% of men under the age of 60 diagnosed with prostate cancer have the less aggressive type; the remaining 1% have the aggressive type of which I have. It is assumed that, once detected, you don't worry too much because chances are you will have the slower-moving type. But what about the other 1%? It seems that it is just plain bad luck. I think I got the short straw!

Jason

Jason lived with his son and his son's family near the coast. He was so enthusiastic about telling his story that he wanted to start the moment I arrived. I overcame this by telling a little about my research while I was setting up the recording equipment and trying to establish a rapport. Jason was 69 at the time of the interview.

Spiritual and religious basics

I am in my high 60s and I've done everything right throughout my life. I'm a Catholic. I go to Church at Christmas and Easter but that's about it. All my family have grown up in the Catholic faith. They have gone to Catholic schools and so have my grandchildren. I'm religious and believe in spirituality.

Frustrations

But, with my story, I'm very annoyed about the whole process. I guess misinformation could be a word. Probably for the last 10 years I've been aware of the word "cancer". I've been doing the PSA. I've been doing the cholesterol and I've been doing the digital, and all that. It's all been fine, 1.9 on the scale of things, all been fine, OK. About nine months ago I thought I'd better do a bowel check as suggested by the TV ads. So I went to the chemist and paid the $15, got the bowel screen check, did the stool sample, sent it away, and it came back OK. I thought, well, that's good. Now for some reason I went to another one a few months later. In the meanwhile I had blood in the bed, blood in the bed. Yes, my second stool sample came back OK. In the meantime I went to a doctor for the blood in the bed. Not my family doctor because I had changed addresses. So I went through the process of having a bowel test so I had a referral to a private hospital for a colonoscopy with Dr Fry. The doctor said, "Well, you're OK in that department but what you need is a prostate check, now!" With that I went to a public doctor – I'm only a pensioner; I'm not on private healthcare cover. I got a referral to a urologist, Dr Edmed. After doing the digital examination he immediately said, "Yes, you are positive". So I was listed in the hospital scheme of things and I waited and waited to get an appointment. I was trying to get an appointment and, in desperation, after 4 to 6 weeks I became very aggressive about it. So I wrote a long letter to the Health Minister. I said, "This is not good enough" and other things; "I just want an appointment. Prostate does kill. I just want a time. I don't care if it's six months but just give me an appointment, not a maybe some time". His secretary replied next day and I got an official letter three days later saying that things are happening but are a bit slow in the hospital system.

"What?"
I was sent to a private hospital to accelerate the process – excellent doctors and nurses – where they took a biopsy. Seven of the eight nodules were contaminated. What? I was then referred back to the hospital scheme of things, and they said, "OK, this is what you do". Being a public hospital patient, you are still under the guidance of a urologist, whatever. I got a CT scan and it did show up positive. The cancer had progressed into my bones and upwards. Then I had to wait another couple of weeks for another CT scan, a bit higher this time, and it did show scatterings in the lung. Wow, that's a knock in the face! So, armed with all this evidence, I went back to the hospital again on appointments. It wasn't too bad considering, once it started, it really did flow. It just took a long time to get started. That was my single biggest problem. So when it got started, there was a guy there, very good. I'd seen a few doctors over the times. They were only juniors but very versed in knowledge with the back-up of the local urologist. Well, this Dr Williams said, "We can't give you radiation because it's progressed. We can't give you chemo either because it's progressed too far; an operation is out of the question. You'll still have some sexual functions, maybe". An important part of my life is sexual function, really.

What are the options?
Anyway, what happened was that I was one of the unlucky ones with high testosterone. It had slipped through the radar. It didn't show up on all the PSA ratings like 2, 5, 8, 12, 15 or higher, it just didn't show up; it was just normal, normal, normal, normal. So I had no warning. So they said, "Well, it's progressed too far", and I said, "What options have I got?", and they said, "The only option you've got is hormone treatment". So I said, "What does this involve – how often, every month, two months …?" and he said,

"Every three months. I'll give you a script, you take it to your chemist, then take it to your local GP and he'll give you an injection in the butt". And I said, "Is that it?" and he said, "Well, that's it!" I said, "Well, can't I do anything else?" and he said, "No. No. See you in three months. It was confirmed with the urologist". "Are you sure that's it?" "Yes, sure, that's it." So, I'll be disillusioned if that's it! My three months is coming up in three or four weeks. I've got to get a PSA to go along with that. Whether it shows anything or not, who knows! I don't know. They'll make a decision on all that. I do feel OK in my body but my mind is a bit screwed up.

Simple "signs"

But a couple of points come to mind. For years I've had an itchy sensation down below. Some people call them crabs or something else but I don't even know that word. Sometimes you scrub yourself in the shower and it's still there. It's an internal sort of thing and you always find that they happen in different places – down below, front and rear. And for years, three or four years I've been asking the local doctor "What's this? Can I get some creams or this or that?" "No, you've got nothing there." One doctor said, "If you think there's something, get some sticky tape on it and we'll examine it". But that wouldn't do any good because it's internal.

But my partner then, well, she had cancer the same year. She had breast cancer. She said, "On reflection now, I've had an itchy nose for the last couple of years. Internal. You can't scratch it." Maybe that's some little sign. If someone had said to me, some smart doctor, or someone, like I'm saying to you now, hey, you don't know, just a wild shot here but how about having a scan done, or something else. This may be a prelim. to something.

So I'm glad you are here to document this because, maybe other people …
I spoke to some of the cancer support people and said, "Hey, guys, have any of you had a sensation down there or around, do you …?" "As a matter of fact, we have." No, no doctor told me this.

"Mandatory tests"

On reflection, a couple of years ago maybe, I would have had a scan or biopsy or whatever. Now, my son is faced with the same scenario. He's 40-

and-a-bit. It's inherent. My mum died of a cancerous thing as well – in the stomach. So he's in line to progress on from me. I said, "It's mandatory, mate, that you get these biopsies done, and colonoscopies". One guy at a workshop a few weeks ago, he stood up and he said, "Is there any man here who hasn't had a colonoscopy in the last year?" Anyway, a few put their hand up and he said, "The rest of you are bloody crazy. Every man our age has got to have a colonoscopy, or a biopsy, and/or other tests." The PSA and the digital is the only one they've got and it's not good enough. There's the progressive side of it.

An emotional road

After being at support groups it was recommended that I see a nurse at another private hospital. Very, very good; highly recommended. She deals in basically erectile dysfunction. All these new words I'm learning – pelvic exercises, outercourse, and others – no doctors told me these words. I've got a lot of information in books. Some I've pushed aside, others are quite relevant. I even pushed some on to my son last night. I haven't had sex really since I've started hormone treatment and that bothers me a lot. I have no urge and definitely no length.

My partner I had before has left me. She had cancer. I tried to follow her through hers but she said I was never her "light", so anyway. She said, "What comes around goes around". Oh, thanks a lot. So I am so fortunate with another lady now who is really, really on side with me. She knows what's happening exactly, precisely. She's offered to come with me next time at a counselling session. I suggested it but she said, "I was going to ask you the same thing". So we have the same thoughts. There were eight or nine couples there at the last prostate support meeting. It was so good to see.

I get quite teary now. I can watch a movie I've watched before with no effect, but now, something happens – the female hormones must kick in, I don't know. All of a sudden the tears are streaming out of my eyes. I don't know what this is. Hot flushes – I haven't had a lot but I have experienced them.

Alternative medicine

I'm on alternative medicine – pawpaw or papaya leaves. I've been reading up about this. I've got on to the internet and I belong to a men's group called "Men's Shed". There's about a hundred people who are fairly active in it and we get to talk. This is fantastic because guys can talk to guys. There are two there coming out of prostate cancer. Men our age can just get together and talk to each other and, if they want to, they can build something. They mightn't have a garage at home – they might be in a high-rise. It's very important for men to get together and chat and you just get to build things. All the tools are there and if you build something it costs $2 for that day for private projects. They build all sorts of things – wooden ducks, horses and toys for the community or charity, so we're actively trying to help these men with something to do. And you get to talk.

I put a sign up saying that I wanted some pawpaw leaves. I've read up about this and I said, "That's for me". So I talk to people and they say, "Yes, I've got some pawpaw leaves, I'll bring some round" or "Come round and we'll get them" and all this. So, I'm into pawpaw leaves. I cut them up. I squash them up. The first lot there were a couple of spiders in there but that's OK – a bit of fresh meat doesn't matter; it's all good! So I cook these things up for two hours, strain it off and get the juice. I'm drinking about 500 or 600 mls per day. I make a couple of 2-litre bottles. This gives me something to do; it gives me a purpose. I feel I'm actively doing something over and above, and instead of, "Well, come back and see me in three months", I'm doing something there. It's good for my mind and it's good for my body. Well, I'm not sure about my body, but I believe it's going to help me. I really believe this. I believe it so strongly, spiritually and otherwise; this is my little grasp on things. I don't pray a lot but I try and meditate. On these pawpaw leaves – I believe it will cure me. I've got people looking for me. They drive along the street and say, "There's some pawpaw leaves over there. I'll take the number down". I'll call them later and have a look. A couple of times I've asked guys and they've said, "Why, are you doing a cook-up, are you?" But I'm certainly aware that it may have some benefits.

Family-based spirituality

I've always been a 100-mile-an-hour guy. I'm a go, go, go guy. I'm an engineer by trade. I've travelled the world a fair bit; I've seen a lot. I've seen half of my own country. I thought work was more important than family. But it's not. In fact, it's very second rate to family. I'm now staying with my son here. He said, "Dad, come and stay with us while we sort this out". So I'm doing that. I believe in God. I believe in spirituality. My family and grandkids are my spirituality.

Personal spirituality

I believe it's a thought. It's a future for me. I can pray for myself. I don't get down and kneel but I certainly believe in the Lord. I know this helps me. I don't think, why is it me? Why me? I don't think that. It's happened and it's happened. I will get on with my cure.

I just think that out there there's some other being. There's a lot of things out there and spirituality is one of those things. I've been reading about well-being and relaxation and I can't quite relax properly. I'm still geared up. But, in my own mind, if I go hard and fast … the problem won't go away but I won't think about it too much. I'm on a regime now with a medical lady at a fitness centre. I go this afternoon to do the first exercises and weights. I would like God to help me. I know God can't heal everybody but I can put myself out there for Him to look down upon me and give me some reason to live. I've been healthy all my life. It's just this last "little speed bump" in my life. I'm not a sick person. I'm reasonably healthy and reasonably fit. So as far as a lot of intensive spirituality – I'm not. I'm not. I've got thoughts that the pawpaw leaves will guide me and God will guide me. I don't pray at night much. I watch a good Catholic movie sometimes. I would like to go to church more often but I don't. I feel life hasn't passed me by. I've had a good life. I've had a good life more than most, actually. I've seen a lot of the world. I've been to India; I've been to the Shah's palace in Iran. I've been to a lot of places. I've been an engineer. It's so great that Australia is Australia. It's just nice to get back to Australia. When you look at what's been happening overseas. Recently a company has gone broke. They employed over 10,000 people; they paid 10 bucks a day and then they skipped off with all their passports.

I mean … that's pretty rough; we are still lucky in Oz. And, I've been given a figure … my Gleason score is 9, which is right up there.

I've turned to a computer to occupy myself and I'm into playing around with these dating sites. People come up; I have a little chat. So I feel there is something else. This will take me through, and other things. Now I'm with a special lady at the moment and she says, "No more coffees". She is right. We give ourselves a very good chance of being happy together. Seriously. She's still working for a couple of years. She's a kindergarten teacher and we go away together. In fact we're going away this weekend. She understands erectile dysfunction but we will work through this. A man loses a lot, particularly in the mind, when this occurs.

More lifts
Well, I like boating. Boating is a big part of my life. I say I have a boating attack. If I can't use my boat at least once in a month, I get depressed. I walk to the beach or go and see some boats. That lifts my spirit. It makes me feel good.

I'm still a believer. I believe in God and say my prayers. In fact, my family and I discussed it last week when we saw "disciple birds" around at a dam while we were fishing. There are always 12 or 13 of them. There are a number of things that lift me. I see the pawpaw leaves as a tool and I believe that, with J.C., and my family, they will guide me through this. The pawpaw is pretty horrible stuff – a bit like Kava. Some people say Aloe vera juice is good. I've given it to a few of my mates and they say, "No! No!" … But I just drink it. It'll get me through this. I don't really feel that if I went to church it would cure me, but I am an optimist – it can only help. I still believe in God.

Also my family lifts me greatly. I live for my family. They don't quite know that. They've always said, "Dad, you must come around more". So that is my spirituality as a rule. I had a partner for seven or eight years on and off, and we had a bit going. That's all gone now, which is a shame because maybe we could have made it. It was just the little things, not the big things that cause the problems. This will never happen again. One must love and be loved back equally.

It was seven months ago that I was directly diagnosed as having advanced prostate cancer – straight off. Boom! And that was because I pushed the issue. No one suggested there were high PSA readings or digital, saying, "Hey, let's check!" And I just thought, well, some blood in the bed, that sort of kicked things off, then the bowel scan. I didn't know anything about the prostate. Everything seemed OK.

Annoyances

I've been annoyed with a few things in my life. My dad died of war wounds. I thought things would have been much better. He was a normal bloke – drank and smoked. He went to the war and come back as a Baptist and gave to the Church 25% of his salary. I followed in his footsteps as being religious, even though I was a Catholic. I thought that things may have been different in life if he'd been around. I'm here for my son now. He has a small business and his wife has her small business. Together they try to make it all happen. It will happen.

Showing spirituality

Well, I don't go to church very much. I haven't been for quite a while. I still respect J.C. I still believe that there is a high power out there. There has to be. We were created for a reason. I've always wanted to do something, to change the world. And I have. I put together my own company. I travelled the world. I invented a product that was quite unique and it's still being used now. I stepped away from it 13 years later. So, in fact, I have done something to change the world in my own little style. I'm still after the magic widget – an inventor with no money to promote.

Over the last few months my spirituality has definitely increased. Through God, doctors, hospitals and injections, family and pawpaw leaves, I believe this will happen. I know people who are relying on other medications, $400 a week or something. I can't afford that. I chose God and the pawpaw leaves to lead me through.

Different avenues for support

I didn't need any support initially. I've received support from a couple of groups of men who have advanced prostate cancer. Some of these groups are up to 100 people. I've come away feeling, "Wow, I'm not alone in this journey". I didn't need any support initially but I'm now very, very grateful for what's there. I now need all the help I can get. Sex has been a big part of my life, but reading books and hearing discussions in the men's group when men talk about sex, they say they are closer now to their partners, even though they do not have a sexual function or can't do it properly. They are closer spiritually and in mind and comfort to each other. A few men in the men's group have a problem and it's also in the books and magazines I'm reading. There are a few good ones around that I'm reading – *Coping With Cancer, Localised Prostate Cancer* … They're excellent. They say the same thing. I'm trying to deal with this because I feel I'm no longer a man. I just can't get it up. They call it "erectile dysfunction"; they have a name for everything. I have now realised that life has more relevance.

My spirituality has a role in helping me cope with my illness because it's been the whole package that has come together. I believe this. Talking with people … there are other aids to being close, there's tablets, there's Viagra, injections. For a man, you lose your manhood. You lose your esteem. I'm in tears talking about it. There's all these books I can get. Some are relevant, some are not.

"Added value"
One of the main things I wanted to add was that I want to document about this itching and irritating. No one had ever said anything about this to me before. If we can document it and a few doctors know about it, maybe someone will say, "Well, maybe it is a precursor to something". And I just want you to document the pawpaw tree leaves. I know that U.S. and British medical companies cannot isolate or patent its benefits properly. How they can help, tie it in with J.C. and spirituality. There have been instances where it has cured people but it hasn't been documented properly. I mentioned this to my local GP. He's broad-minded enough to see that it may help, or at least for my mind. If I can help, and people can relate to something I've said, and they get cured, well, the world's set on fire; cancer might just be a word.

Stephen

Stephen lived in a resort complex near the ocean. He was keen to explain the reason that he had volunteered to be a participant in the study because he believed he had benefited considerably from his personal experiences in spiritual development. He had tried many ways to approach his illness and eventually found the approach that was suiting him. He was 67 at the time he told his story.

The beginning of the physical journey ...

It started six years ago. I had a busy legal practice in Brisbane and what was happening was that I had tried to ease off a bit and we bought this house and worked in Brisbane for four days and came down here for Friday, Saturday and Sunday and I played golf. I was really putting six days' work into four. Prior to that I was really working six and seven days a week. I was really working hard and my wife was working in the business as well. But that was OK. I had high blood pressure and high cholesterol but I'd been on medication for that for 30 years. I thought I had a heart attack a few years ago but it wasn't; it was just that my blood pressure was high. But really, my other health was OK. One thing that was happening was that my sexual activity was declining but when you go to the doctor he just says, oh, I'll just give you some Viagra or something; you know they never really ... you know ... So this was happening but no one was really ... you know, the prostate thing never came up. No one ever suggested that there might have been a prostate problem or doing anything about it. I was having a PSA test in with my cholesterol but everyone was watching my cholesterol more than the PSA. I wasn't even conscious of what a PSA was. I mean, that was the most shocking thing, it wasn't on the radar. No one ever mentioned to me that you are going to get prostate cancer.

So, I was coming down and playing golf and all of a sudden I started to get some bone pain in my legs. So I went to the physiotherapist – blah, blah, blah – I'd go away. I stopped playing golf and then it came back again so I went back to the physio. So this went on and off, then, all of a sudden, one day it didn't go away.

... and the spiritual journey

Talking about spirituality, I went to a funeral of one of my clients, and, at the funeral, my legs started to become really sore. We went to the wake and then it seemed someone was telling me that something was wrong with me. I think it was funny that it started at a funeral and this time it didn't go away. It became very bad on the weekend; I might have taken some Panadol or something. It got worse so I went back to my doctor and he said straight away, "You'd better go and see a bone specialist". I had an appointment in the next few days and I told the guy my symptoms. He tried to move my legs around and he said, "Gee, you might need a hip replacement" and I said "That's pretty scary". Anyway, he said, "Go and get an x-ray straight away" so I did an x-ray and I came back to him and he said, "No, it's not that, it's something else". And he was thinking, and he said, "You'd better go and get an MRI". So he arranged for this and referred me to a bone guy. All this was just happening. One good thing – I was privately insured and I wasn't jerked around by the medical profession. A lot of people take six months to get diagnosed. Within a week I had all the tests and they found that I had an enlarged prostate. They saw that I hadn't had a PSA test for a while. The last one I'd had it was 3 and then within two years it was 24. I'd missed the test I was supposed to have. I'd just forgot about having it. Before that the guy had rung me up when he'd got the MRI results and said, "You've got something on your bone". He called me in and he said, "Look, I'll give you a scan. You might be lucky, you might just have prostate cancer – a secondary". He referred me to a prostate cancer guy. In the meantime they did a biopsy and found that it wasn't bone cancer, it was prostate cancer in the bone, a secondary which is bad enough. Then I got shovelled from one guy to another and the last guy I saw was a urologist and, like the oncologist, he said it was incurable – blah, blah, blah – so within the space of a week ...

Feeling like ...

I felt like ****! I mean, I'm thinking, I'm going to die. I mean, they said they could treat it but not cure it and everyone is sticking their finger up my bum, and you know … And I thought, this is ridiculous, how can it be happening? I've got cancer; I'm supposed to die of a heart attack. By this time they're talking about something I've never known about, know nothing about … By the time you get to see the urologist – he's the last guy – they've already worked out what it was and he said, "Well, you've done a biopsy and it's confirmed; the Gleason score is a 4 plus 4, which is not the worst but is not good, together with a PSA of 24 – it's in the bone already". I must admit that the bone pain had gone up so I took some Voltarin so that did help. It wasn't that big – they'd picked it up early. So I said, "What are my options?" and he said, "Well, you've got no options – you can have a hormone injection or nothing". That was it. So, what do you do? Just have a hormone injection – bang.

So the hormone injection dropped it down from 24 to 1.7, then it went to 1.0, and it didn't go much lower than that. So that sort of worked.

All the side-effects – "that stuff"

So I had all the side-effects – the hot flushes, the memory thing, the depression – all that stuff was going on and I had a busy practice. I've got people ringing me up for advice about all sorts of things every day and I've got two offices and I think I can't … you know … I can't do this. Eventually, it kills you. The doctor says you don't know how long it's going to last. The hormones only last for so long. It slows the cancer growth but after that it will start growing again. After that, there's not much at that stage you can do. You can have some chemotherapy that can have a small benefit. You get bone pain, and you take pain-killers … It's not much of a prognosis, so I'm thinking, I don't see much point in working anymore, so, I'm thinking (I didn't even consult my wife), I said, "I'll put the practice on the market". So we sold one fairly easily – the best part. The other one I kept for six months and just kept on running that. Then I had a disability policy that would pay until I was 65 and I was 62. It paid $4,000 a month. So we had enough money. We were reasonably comfortable. We were self-funded retirees so we didn't have any pension. So I sold both practices for a reasonable price. So that was good. If I had to work I could have but I thought, if I've only got a few years to go, I may as well enjoy it, so what the heck! I'm 67 now and this started in 2005 so it's been six years. I was thinking about retirement but I was just a workaholic and we were making good money. So that all happened, and we decided to sell everything up. Bingo!

Spiritual development

What happened in the meantime, the Thailand thing came up and I'll just explain what happened there. We worked in Thailand back in the 70s. We lived there in Bangkok for two years. I worked with a big company there and it nearly killed me, but I was young and silly. We left there and didn't go back for 25 years. Anyway, before I was diagnosed, we had collected enough frequent flyer points to travel Business Class somewhere. So, we'd been working our guts out and decided to close the office for two weeks. So we decided to go to Chiang Mai (North Thailand) – we hadn't been there for a long time. So we booked the tickets. Then, six months later, before I was diagnosed, we were at a party and we were talking to someone who had been to some resort in Chiang Mai – some health resort – and he said we should go there. That sounded interesting so I talked to my wife – she's into health stuff; I'm not into anything natural – I'm straight down the line. So we decided to Google it and found out the things they did – it was a Tao centre and they taught Tai Chi, Qi Gong and all that stuff. I booked in for a few days and thought we might then go somewhere else. So, I get diagnosed in August and we're going there in December.

So I'm thinking I might need this for myself now so we might spend the whole time there. So we sold one part of the business and we get there and stay there and we start doing all this stuff – meditation, massages, Qi gong and others; so we started doing all this stuff and you get up in the morning and start doing these exercises and breathing and – blah, blah, blah – you know, a lot of stuff, and they say if you do this every day you can live to be a hundred. And then they start saying you can start strengthening the lungs by internal means – not, like, running around the block – and also the liver, your bones, and I'm thinking, this cancer is going to get into all these places, maybe … maybe I can do something about it. It started me thinking – the doctors are not going to cure me; they've given me a bit of time – all they've done is bought me some time – so I've got to work out what am I going to do with the time I've got. I could just sit around and have some red wine every night, do nothing and get fat, but I might as well do something about it. The stuff I was doing at the resort all started to make sense; this was the first time I had a bit of hope. I didn't quite know how I was going to do it. It wasn't a cure hope; it wasn't going to be hard work, that I had to "do this" , do it every day – blah, blah, blah – it's not praying to a god or anything, it's really bringing energy from the universe into your body and all this stuff.

The beginnings of change

At this time I'm still pretty depressed. The side-effects of the drugs – I couldn't think; you go from having a normal testosterone down to nothing – you know, you're feeling like ****. But I started to change. We were staying in a town house for two weeks and then we found out that all the places there we could buy. They were all owned by people and then they rent them out. Then we found out the guy who owned the house we were in wanted to sell – US$130,000. So I'm thinking, if I need to do this practice I've got to come over here a lot. So we thought – we had the money anyway – so we could buy the house and rent it out. It wasn't a particularly good investment except it would be for my health. Maybe it would help me live a bit longer. So we came home, thought about it, went back again and did the deal – we bought the place and we've had nearly 20 visits. We've been to other places – Europe and so on – but that's all we do now. We go two or three times a year to Thailand. The reason we do it is that there is a guru there. He runs a training place. The training lasts five weeks, twice a year, so we always go – there's one in July/August and one in January/February. Sometimes we do the course and sometimes we just spin off the courses. You pay some extra money and go there in the morning and do some meditation and there's extra stuff that's on what you can do. So that's what we started to do and that's all it really was, but it really was something that I decided to do, to make the effort to make myself fit and healthy. That was the best advice my urologist said. I said, "What can I do to live longer?" and he said, "Well, all I can say is that there is a lot of other stuff that people go on with and talk about – food, vitamins, magic cures, but if you keep yourself fit and healthy you've got more chance". I think I know now what being fit and healthy means. It's not that easy when the drugs are working against you but I thought I'd go to Thailand and try to turn my head around. So that was the first turning of my head. That gave me a bit of optimism. So, of the six years, that was probably what I call stage one of my life. It was going to Thailand and doing stuff there.

Treatments – more "stuff"

As I came into stage two, my PSA had dropped from 24 and settled down around the 1 mark; it went down and came up a bit occasionally. Some guys try to get it right down. They make a big thing of getting it down to zero but I read all the stuff about having more drugs. I was having monotherapy – one injection; other people have many things – triple androgen. I have it every six months. I have a drug called Eligard – one of the newer ones, and maybe I was lucky about that. So I have it every six months – used to have it every three but it doesn't really matter whether it is six or seven months. It's not going to make any difference. So that's kept my PSA down around the 1 mark. Sometimes it goes up and down a little bit but I seem to be able to turn it down. I go back to Thailand and do a lot of stuff. I had acupuncture. I wasn't doing much meditation at this stage but I seemed to be able to turn it down when I had to turn it down. What you've got to avoid is this PSA thing. It can get out of hand, then it's really hard to knock this back. You can't ever let it go. So I reckon, from all I've read, I just have to keep my PSA under control.

More frequent meditation

So the next stage I really got into meditation. I did a little bit up in Thailand but I eventually got to a camp (back in Australia) that was mainly for women with breast cancer. So I went there but thought it wouldn't be much because it was really for women. (I went to a support group once for men – supporting each other. I gave my story and I was feeling pretty good but then all the other men started moaning and groaning. They were talking about their chemotherapy and all that stuff. All they wanted to do was tell their story; they weren't interested in my story. They sucked all the energy out of me and I didn't have enough to share so I didn't go back. I'm OK in myself but I can't support anyone else; I just haven't got enough strength.)

So I'd been to the camp once and I decided to go back there again to do some meditation. So I started doing some of this and I found it very hard. And then they said that they were having a retreat and that they'd like me to come – they needed some men. So after some umm-ing and ah-ing I decided to go. There were three guys there and, to me, I was really the only normal man there. Anyway, there were nine women there telling their stories and I'm there telling my story. After hearing theirs, I thought, I'm lucky. They're all females and they had their problems – their husbands had left them or their kids hated them, they're struggling with their chemo, they've got all these treatments, they're taking this and that, they've got no money; and I'm thinking, I'm not complaining. I reckon my cancer had a worse prognosis than all of theirs but I'm doing better. So that was a real turning point, realising that I'm doing better than I should be for whatever reason, so I started to do a lot more meditation.

I made some good friends out of that. We talk about connection. I made a good connection with a woman there. She was crook at the time but she's OK now. But all this meant that I felt I want to help these people. I felt I had something to give.

I got more into meditation. About this time my PSA jumped from about 1.1 to 1.8. That was a big shock. I don't know what happened. I thought, maybe there's some reason … This changed me a bit, like emotionally. A few things happened which affected me. I don't know why it happened but it did. I was able to get it back again. It has jumped again. I did a test the other day. It's 2.4 now. I was a bit unwell; I had a virus and my brother was sick so I think that affected me. My doctor's not worried about it. It does jump a bit but in my mind I can turn it around again.

With all of this you can do things with your mind. From that time of meeting new people and talking with them, I started to get insights into people's mind. Like, all of a sudden, people started talking to me. All sorts of people would talk to me about all their problems. People would spill their hearts to me and tell me everything. All of a sudden I could understand relationships for the first time in my life – love and friendships all that kind of stuff.

"Feeling" experiences

The other thing was that I did have a treatment with a shaman. Back in Thailand. This guy did some exorcism on me. It did have an impact on me because what he kept saying to me was, "What do you feel, what do you feel?" From that time, I did feel things. I feel a lot more than I ever did. I think differently about relationships and am more conscious of this. Maybe it's because of the low testosterone I have that makes me think more like a female maybe, or something like that.

My attachment to a female friend was part of it. That was a bit unexpected so that might have had something to do with it. But the meditation seemed to help; it seemed to be part of it but maybe this was a way of dealing with it. The shaman, meditation and the attachment all helped a bit.

Substance of meditation

I do three lots of meditation really. I do meditation in camp which is more mindfulness, which is really, you know, guided meditation, breathing or counting or something like that, or sometimes going down and sitting in a cave. Basically, sometimes it's guided – you must be going down a hill, sitting in a cave or sitting on a beach or something like that. That's interesting but I don't do it that much. Maybe it can work. It's mainly just calming your mind and trying to keep yourself quiet; just not thinking about anything. It's really like a half-sleep; I did some yesterday.

Then there's Zen meditation – totally silent – where you sit and do nothing; try not to think at all. There are different techniques. They say don't think, don't do anything; you've just got to sit there for 20 minutes. You don't say anything. What are you going to do? You can count; you can breathe. There are different forms of meditation. I just think that the basic thing is that it calms you down and it has a good effect on you. It actually improved my golf game – which is quite amazing. It made me play better golf even though I'm not a great golfer. I seem to be able to do it when I want to. I'm not a great meditator but it's giving more calmness. I don't do much at home but I do it twice a week at another place; I mean, you're supposed to do it every day. I do listen to meditative music at night and in the morning.

Mindfulness is a general meditation with some guidance. The man we go to does some of this but he is more into Zen which is total silence and breathing. I don't relate to that so much.

My spiritual background

Just looking at the religious side (I know that's not the whole thing), I was raised an Anglican and went to Sunday School until I was an older boy and all that stuff. Now I'm not a disbeliever, I'm probably a believer but I don't go to church or anything like that. Thailand is Buddhist. It's a nice religion and we've been to a lot of Buddhist stuff but I don't see myself as a Buddhist, although I've taken on board some Buddhism. I feel comfortable in that sort of environment but I've never bothered to practise it too much. Buddhism is a nice thing to have in Thailand because when you go to a Buddhist thing it's very peaceful and things like that. The Dao stuff is Chinese-based, of course, and, while they do have symbols and all that, it's really not a "god" thing. You're halfway to god but you don't pray for him to help. If you want to be cured, you've got to do it yourself and look after your own body. If you want to be cured and have a long life, it's hard work and a healthy life and you can do all these practices. This is the thing that has resonated with me. I guess the Dao practice is a form of religion. The other thing is helping people. I do find myself helping cancer patients although sometimes it has a negative effect on me. Somehow I've developed some spirituality, whatever that is …

Getting a lift – "I can do it"

If I want to, I can lift myself above but I've got to want to do it. If I want to manipulate my PSA, I can do it. If you want to lift yourself up to shoulder height, you can. The hardest thing is staying there. I think that's why some religious gurus get up there and stay there. Before, I didn't know there was an "up there" sort of thing. The hardest thing is finding the focus to let you do it. And, I want to get there and stay there.

Using my spirituality

Well, it comes down to where you are with your life. We all have certain routines but I want to spend time with people who care. I'm choosy about how I spend my time; that's the important thing. Sometimes I play golf with a guy who is also unwell but he's OK, he's not a drainer. I try to avoid the sorts of people who drain your energy and have a negative effect on you. You have to keep away from those sorts of people. It can knock you around too much otherwise.

I think it's a matter of focussing. I use my PSA as a guide because that's the only thing I've got. I've just got to keep that under control and when it goes up a bit I don't necessarily do more things but I focus more on what I'm doing. It's really getting my head around it. I think the secret is it's your head. If my head's right, I'm OK, but people sometimes disrupt it or upset you. The other thing is that because of the drug I'm on – I mean, I have no testosterone – the side-effects of what I'm doing – it's been a long time – six years – you get depression, you get emotional. I mean, this emotional thing can be caused by the drug – and there's memory loss, depression; a lot of what I am doing is counteracting the effects of the drug. That brings you back to normal, so you can live a normal life. But what I'm doing focusses your mind – it's a bit like when I saw my brother and I thought, "I'm not going to finish up like that". I thought, "That could be me in five years' time". I'm not going to sit around waiting to die. I've got to find another way around it. Sometimes you do feel you can't do something – well, what's the point of this?; it would be easier not to be here. No one really cares, or ... but they really do care, but ... you know what I mean. I guess you are more sensitive ...

Sometimes I wonder if I should have given up work or not. I couldn't have done it in the first couple of years but lately I've wondered. It's not that I miss the work but I miss the contact with people; but in my case, I had to do what I had to do.

Special points along the journey
Recognising the Tao system of spirituality was the first point on my journey. The second was with the camp retreat where we had the discussions with other cancer patients. That triggered other things and enhanced my spirituality. That changed me as well. I've had little changes up and down since then.

A couple of other things. Golf is important to me. When I was first diagnosed, I just couldn't concentrate. The secret of golf is concentrating and focussing and I couldn't. I was up and down. One of the things that has come out of my calmness is some extraordinary moments on the golf course where I've done some great things. I don't know why or how; they've just happened, especially when I've come back from Thailand and that's more of a focussing. It's a calmness and focussing on the course. If I can go around the course calm, I know I'm in good shape. Now I know that if I can play good golf, I know my health's good.

The other thing I've gone back to is music. My mum was a good musician. She was a classical pianist. I had a few lessons but she taught me how to play rock'n'roll chords and things like that. I did play in a band when I was at university. That was something I always enjoyed. I drifted away from that and now I've just gone back to it. I bought a keyboard and I'm learning again, so that's something that's important. That's something I'm obviously going to keep pursuing and developing.

I think that playing golf in a nice, calm way – to me it's not so much that I'm playing a good game but it's that I'm at peace with myself and I keep thinking that if I can do that I'm physically OK. I can walk around the golf course and come back very tired, as I was yesterday after 18 holes. At one time I didn't have the energy to walk around the course. But now, it's not just the enjoyment, but it's my mental state. It's more than just playing golf. I know that if I can do that I'm OK.

"Keep your head around it all"
The only other thing I want to add is that I went to a doctor and discussed healthy living with him. That's the thing that you get off the track with. I really need to do some focussing on what I'm eating. That's all you can do except keep your head around it all.

Alan

Alan had a long cancer journey. Some of the circumstances in the weeks prior to the interview were also traumatic for him in that his immediate family had been affected by the Queensland floods. He demonstrated his ability to adapt to the circumstances. We met in a guesthouse common living room as he was having treatments and living away from home. His usual home was in a country town some 350 kilometres from Brisbane. At the time of the interview he was 63.

The start of prostate cancer

Well, I'm 63 and I had an abnormal reading way, way back. I was officially diagnosed over seven years ago. First of all I had a scare – I had a thyroid growth; they couldn't find out whether it was benign or whether it wasn't. They took the growth and some of my thyroid out and decided it was benign. So after that the doctor said, "I'd better do a test to see if you are coping with half a thyroid. I'll give you a PSA test too". When he did that, it came up as 13 or something. I had the test several years before but the doctor said, "It's a little bit above average. We'll have to keep an eye on it". In that intervening time I'd gone through a marriage break-up, divorce and that sort of thing, and the last thing you are doing is going to the doctor for a PSA test. There are that many other things going on. It just got away from me, I guess. By the time I was diagnosed it was up around 17.2. The urologist said there was about a 35% chance that if we do take the prostate out we will get a cure. So I thought, 35% is better than nothing so I'll go with that. So they did, and, with much persistence, I actually spoke with the person who reported on the outcome of the surgery. He said that the cancer was within 0.4 of a millimetre of the outer casing of the gland. So it was still within and they considered it still local.

Communication difficulties

That was quite an episode in itself because I rang up and asked to speak to the doctor who wrote the report. The receptionist said, "No, no, I can't give you that information – confidentiality ..." and all this sort of stuff. "If you want to know anything about that, you'll have to ask your GP and he'll have to talk to the reporting doctor to find out what the answer is." I said, "No, it's my report, I'm entitled to know what the report is". I kept ringing up until I got a different receptionist and she put me through to the doctor that signed the report. He came on the phone. He was very good; he talked about everything I wanted to know. He kept saying, "Is there anything else that you want to know before I hang up?" He answered everything I wanted. That's how persistent you've got to be to get the information you want. They pull this "privacy" on you because in many cases they are just too lazy to have to do anything.

Biopsy trauma – "I tell you what ..."
When I did the needle biopsy before the prostatectomy, they told me you had no feeling in the prostate and that anaesthetics wouldn't do any good, but, I tell you what, one of the biggest lies that can be told is that you have no feeling in the prostate. Other fellas have said that they had an anaesthetic when they had theirs done. It shouldn't be done without anaesthetic. But after the third needle you are that bruised you don't feel that much.

Consequences of surgery
After I had the prostatectomy, I had a lot of trouble with incontinence for about eight months. I got on to a doctor who was a physiotherapist and who had similar problems. He got on to a heavy exercise program and eventually cured himself so he published this. I spoke to him on the phone several times; I've only met him once. After eight months I got on top of it. I went back to work then and eventually the readings started to rise again. I had bone scans but they couldn't tell me where the cancer was. I went back in three months and had another bone scan and the cancer showed up in four places. Obviously there wasn't enough to show up earlier. The cancer was in the rib, the sternum, shoulder blade and ... probably the other shoulder ... They wanted to put me on Androcur or one of those anti-androgen drugs that suppress the testosterone. I had been on a course of Androcur prior to the surgery because the doctor said it would help control it and shrink the prostate a certain amount and this would make it easier to remove. About four weeks prior to the surgery the PSA dropped down

from 17.2 down to 0.3 or something. So that probably helped me quite a bit, but after the surgery it rose again and, as I said, I got cancer in the bones then.

They wanted to put me back on something like Androcur but I had some of the worst headaches I'd had in my life when I was on Androcur. I had pains in me head – it wasn't like a normal headache where you'd have pain in one part of your head. This one was like having a marble rolling around inside your head where it would move from one part of the head to another, and these were the worst headaches I'd ever had in my life and I wasn't going back there again. So I elected the older type of treatment – a bilateral orchiectomy. That dropped my PSA down for quite a long time but, after 12 months or so, that failed. I then went on to chemotherapy – six months of that – and got quite good results. This then failed and I had to go off that. Meanwhile, I was on steroids while I was on that. I had to have medication while I was taking that because I was having reflux problems – I'd eat something and it would come straight back up.

Trauma of treatment
I wasn't very sick when I was on that chemo. When that finished I went on to something else and that made me sick so I came off that then and I really went downhill. The PSA just kept rising – as far as 6,380 – and I was down to the stage where I would crawl out of bed at 4 o'clock in the afternoon, have a shower, have a bit of tea and go back to bed. That was the limit.

Then I got on to a trial that was run at the Wesley Hospital – MDV 3100 – I had to take four capsules every day. They weren't destructive of the healthy cells but they affected the cancer cells. It was an androgen antagonist that stopped the body producing hormones that the cancer could feed on. I did very well on that and moved away from being virtually bedridden. I got back on my feet and got to the stage where I could get out of bed, get out to service the motor vehicle; I went back to old-time dancing – enough to go dancing 'til midnight of a Saturday night – this sort of thing. This made a marvellous difference. In six months it took my PSA from 6,380 to 640 – a tenth in six months. After that the readings started to rise about 700 a month average. After another three months they took the supply tablets from me because they weren't working. It's climbing again now uncontrollably. I'm looking now at going on to another trial drug that was very similar to the first chemo I went on, maybe in a month's time. At this stage, I probably will refuse it because I will have to go on to a steroid that I was on for 16½ months. This gave me a cushion on the soles of my feet – when you walk you feel as though you're walking on a cushion, which wasn't good for my dancing. It affected my eyes to the extent that I gave up reading; I had trouble reading street signs. I complained about this to the eye specialist and he said, "Oh, it would be the chemo that was doing it". I complained to my oncologist and he said, "No, it would be the steroids that would be doing it. It changes the sodium level in the eyes. It's then not possible to focus sharply". Meanwhile, the cancer's spreading. It's in all my ribs, pelvis and spine, and shoulders. It's now obviously spreading into the femurs because they're aching. And I've had to go on to pain medication to tolerate it.

Juggling

I had to have a blood transfusion yesterday because my creatine readings were too high and I couldn't have Zometa. I've been having this every month ever since I started on chemo to stop the migration of calcium from going from the bones into my bloodstream and clogging up my kidneys and liver. So now it's a case of juggling the pain medication. These things affect your bowels and you finish up with constipation; then you have to take stuff for constipation and you get nauseous and you have to take stuff for that. Every drug causes another complication. There's nothing treating the cancer of the bone. It's all pain management. The PSA readings are now up to 4,930 again, where they were 6,380 last time.

Feelings and emotions

I've isolated myself pretty well. In the last 10 years when my marriage broke up I've lived by myself ever since, pretty well. I've virtually no support from my family. I get a little bit of support from my daughter. She's officially my carer but she's limited to what she can do at the moment because she was affected by the floods in January; she hasn't got a house to live in so I can't stay with her, even though I'm sick – that's why I'm staying in an accommodation lodge while I'm having treatment. She's living in a caravan. The only thing in her house is a toilet and a washing machine. The rest of it is gutted. So she's not in a position to help me.

Spiritual basis

Well, I've always been brought up in a Christian religion. I grew up a Methodist. I voted for the formation of the Uniting Church, which I thought just made sense because there are so many parallel religions. There was really no reason for them to be separate. In some places it has worked; in others it has created four religions instead of three. I'll attend any church that's convenient to me at the time. When I'm visiting one member of my family I'll attend the Church of Christ because it's the only church there. When I'm in another centre, I'll go up the road to the Uniting Church. When I'm at home I go to the Presbyterian Church where other members of my family go. These days I feel that a lot of those churches are very generic. A lot of them do not have full-time ministers that can give you the spiritual support that they used to years ago. At one time you used to have a minister in your town for your religion that you could go to for counselling if you wanted to. These days they're supposed to cover two or three towns so they are never there when you want them. A lot of it is done by lay preachers these days and they just have a series of church services laid out for the year or they go on to the internet and download church services from the internet and you can virtually go to half a dozen different churches. All the services are, as I say, generic. I've got no problem with that, I suppose, but they might celebrate the communion slightly differently. They might have different thoughts on what age a child might be baptised, but you can live with that as long as they follow God the Creator ... I was brought up basically on the Apostles' Creed. "I believe in God the Father, maker of heaven and earth, Jesus Christ His only Son and our Lord, conceived of the Holy Spirit, born of the virgin Mary, suffered under Pontius Pilate, was crucified, dead and buried ..." you've got this summary of the Christian religion. A lot of these religions, you can go along and say, "Yep, I can agree with all that, but we're Presbyterians, we're Church of Christ, Wesleyans or something – but they all agree with that basic creed".

Religious support – "I'd like to sit down and talk ..."

To assist my spirituality I'd like to sit down and talk about where I am at and pray about my future, you know. You either do it yourself or the person you pray with has to be sincere – they're not just a wage-earner; it's not just their job; they've got to be sincere.

I don't find myself involved in a lot of personal spirituality. I do like to go and worship with people. I like to sing, pray, have communion ... fellowship. You've got friends who will sit down and talk with you. This is where this spiritualty as a broad, floating, umbrella sort of thing – I don't really agree with that sort of thing. You get a congregation and within that congregation you do have a real spirituality. You just can't have a floating sort of thing where everyone can have their own spirituality. It's got to have a base on something.

I can sit down with people of many religions and enjoy discussing religious matters. They can be Mormons, they can be ... as long as there is common ground. But I can't sit down with an atheist and have a discussion about spirituality because they don't want to know and they don't understand. They haven't had the education.

Over the period of my cancer journey my spirituality has stayed much the same. Oh, it may have increased a little. The thing is, some people will ask, "How do you cope with it?" and I say, "You get used to it". I mean, I've been living with it that long ... I've counselled a lot of people who have been diagnosed with it or have had members of their families who have been diagnosed. They're just knocked out by the diagnosis and all the treatment they're going to go through. And I say to them, "Look, you do become used to it. You just become used to it after a while. I mean, it's like going to the dentist – you mightn't like going to the dentist, you know you've got to go, and you know it's for your own good that you go so you do it. It's the same thing; you just keep lining up for treatment".

I first started with a support group and they were a great help to me when I was first diagnosed because, when the doctor first tells you it is a cancer, the rest of the conversation is a blur. You don't remember it. I just tell them that that's normal.

The lifts – "you smile all the time"

I used to be in photography a lot but I've lost interest in that. My main interest is old-time dancing. I've always done it; I do a lot of new ones down here. I've been going to dancing down here whenever I come down. I know enough people now that, if I don't know a dance, the ladies are happy to help me learn the dance. It lifts me because of the music. You've got to dance with the music; you've got company and contact. You forget about all your problems; you just concentrate on enjoying the dance. You have a laugh and a joke. One of the ladies said, "You smile all the time", and I said, "When I get it right, I smile; when I get it wrong, I laugh"; so I'm always happy; it doesn't matter.

Spirituality helps – "I'm not scared of dying"
My spirituality helps me a lot. I'm not scared of dying; it's the pain and suffering that worries me. I'm ready to die and any time; that doesn't worry me. I could go to bed tonight and die in my sleep and that would not worry me at all.

I'd like more spiritual support from people close to me, especially in my home town. Nobody wants to get too close to somebody who is going to die, unless they are very rare people. I've got good friends. I've got one in particular at the moment and she said, "It's a pity you're so sick", and I said, "If I wasn't so sick I wouldn't be here, I'd be back at home working." She couldn't accept that. She's a little bit older than me and she's still working; she does nursing, on call. I said, "That's what we do – as long as we're well enough, we work. If we're not well enough, we stop work. If we are too sick to work and too sick to enjoy life, that's the way of our lives; it's silly, but that's what we do".

There was another lady – we're still good friends; she's been a great help to me religion-wise – and everything was fine until it was described to her one day that prostate cancer was acute until the stage where it escapes from the prostate and metastasises to elsewhere in the body when it becomes chronic. That hit her like a ton of bricks and after that she decided she didn't want to be a serious friend any more. She couldn't cope with it. That is the case when you reach this stage – you can't expect anybody to be too close because they know they're going to get hurt.

Ken

Ken lived in a comfortable home near the coast. The interview was carried out in a relaxing environment, in the outdoors, next to his swimming pool. At the time he told his story he was 69.

The beginning of the cancer journey

The early part of the journey started when I had high PSA levels. I was fit and healthy and the GP agreed that I was one of the last people he would expect to see with a problem. After a couple of more PSA and other normal checks and biopsies, it turned out that it was an aggressive cancer and had to be attended to and removed as soon as possible. So the prostate was removed and it was found that the cancer was outside the gland and the post-surgery PSA results weren't good so subsequent radiation pulled things down to a reasonable number for about three months but then it started to sky-rocket again. It was the doubling rate that caused the doctors concern about what to do next. So I then went on to hormone treatment for about two years. That held it at bay for a while. I tried a number of others things: Chinese herbal medicine; and I went on to a trial program with a professor up in Queensland – a melaleuca-based trial. The end result was that after two years the PSA level was rising.

At that stage the doctors were predicting a shorter life-span after I went to an oncologist over 12 months ago, and I was told that it had spread to the bones and there wasn't much they could do for me. They told me to go away and enjoy myself and get my affairs in order and probably by about the middle of 2009 things should go pretty badly by that stage. They didn't say I was going to die by then but they didn't have much hope of me getting beyond that.

The beginning of the spiritual journey

In the meantime, Peter, a friend of my middle son whom I'd met from time to time at various family functions – Christmas and birthdays and things – was a Christian guy. I had as a young fellow been involved in a church but I had an experience with a minister at the time who I thought was a bit of a

Smart Alec. I steered away from that as the result of the couple of experiences and basically left the church alone as a result of it. But when this friend of my son's (Peter) spoke to me one day and said that his father-in-law had contracted prostate cancer – and this fellow asked if I would like to spend a little bit of time with his father-in-law to give me a bit of help and guidance. I did that and then Peter rang up and said, "God has spoken to me and basically He suggested that I talk to you and maybe you might like to come along to our church". It was a really emotional phone call. I'm one who is reasonably strong-willed and strong-minded but I can get emotional like anybody; … that struck a chord with me and I went along to the church. My wife, Sue, was brought up as a Catholic and had traditional upbringings of a Catholic which is something a lot of people aren't comfortable with because it's a bit of fire and brimstone and "repent your sins" type of approach, whereas this church we went along to, which was a non-denominational church – Reach Out for Christ – the guy who was the pastor there had a totally different outlook on preaching the Bible. It was basically built around "Jesus loves you no matter what and he died on the cross for our sins and we can be born again free of sin" and he basically did that for the betterment of our life. I clicked on to this and so did Sue. As an offshoot of this particular church there was another Reach Out for Christ church a few kilometres away. Dr David Mitchell was the preacher there and we went up to what he called his healing Wednesday sessions and that really struck a chord.

This went on for a few weeks and spread into a few months. In the meantime, I had reached the stage where the oncologist said, "Well look, it's in your bones now and you might make it to Christmas 2009; Christmas 2010 I don't like your chances". But I was still feeling OK and still believed I could beat it but what I found was that, as I started to get more and more involved in the church and go back and read the Bible and learn what its teachings and preachings were on a Sunday, Sue and I realised that there were a number of things that happened from the time we made a decision to move from Sydney to come here. These things could not have been just coincidence; they were deemed to happen from a higher order.

Naturopathy

As a result of the things that happened on the way, we came in touch with a naturopath who was from the Seventh Day Adventist group and part of the Christian Naturopathic Association. He came to talk to the group and I liked what he had to say so we went and saw him. His approach to help people with serious health issues (and not so serious health issues for that matter – people might just have digestive problems and things like that) ... his basic teaching was that we came from the dust and basically we should be living a lifestyle where our food source comes from the land. Sue and I always ate fairly well, we thought, but when we got involved with this naturopath, he started to talk about things that coincided with what we were reading as I was making my way through the Old Testament, and I thought, "This is clicking; this is making sense".

The oncologist said at that stage, "You've got what we call headlights – spots in your bones from where the cancer has gotten to – and all we can do is keep zapping these"; and I found out that what they were doing was not curing the cancer but trying to bring the pain level down – but I didn't have any pain.

Coming together

So I put all together what I had learnt from the naturopath, and the reading of my Bible, and what had happened with a number of events that had happened one after the other that caused us to relocate to where we are living now. Had we not come here I would never have come across the church or I would never have come across Peter, the guy who rang me up and said that God had spoken to him. I would never have come across the naturopath.

The naturopath was basically saying that our belief is above all reproach and our lifestyle was needed to be followed in a particularly healthy way with the Bible in the background giving us direction. He made the comment that most people who came to him had difficulty in following the tight regime on lifestyle that he would suggest to us. I know I am strong-willed and I'm not one who follows the general public. I'm a leader, not a follower. You give me a brick wall – I'll knock it down. He said to me, "You are going to have to take this slowly because people often can't handle the regime". I said that I had a lot going for me. I've got God on my side and my wife who really is attuned because of her training in health and she is a great support and what I was getting out of the church was a great support so I said, "Bring it on!"

Anyway, I'd been going to church for about six months, and, after these healing sessions with Dr David Mitchell (each Wednesday he would have healing sessions there for those who had health issues), I'd thought very seriously about becoming a born-again Christian and I went out one day to have hands-on healing from him. And, it's pretty emotional for me right now to think about that day because I felt this warm glow come through my body like I'd never felt before; I knew something had happened and it was really something I had never experienced before. It was very emotional.

Severing ties with the doctor

So I kept going there. I went back to the Wednesday sessions a couple of times. I didn't always go out to the front for the healing. A couple of times I did and each time I could feel this warm glow coming over my body which I could never explain. Anyway, the bottom line was that the doctors said they could do nothing but slow the cancer down but I said, "I'm not about that; I want to cure it". I believe that what I was doing with the naturopath and my approach to believing in God that He would speak to me and keep directing me – Sue and I sat down one day and we said, "We're not going back to the doctors because they said, 'Go away and enjoy yourself; there's nothing we can do for you. We'll just put you on hormone treatment' – that's not going to cure anything; that's just going to slow it down". So I said, "Why go back to get these PSA numbers because they are no absolute guarantee that you've got cancer; all it's going to do is add anxiety". So we made a conscious decision not to go back to the doctor. This was about six months ago.

I've got to the stage where I go to the naturopath and he does live blood cell tests. I first went to him about 18 months ago when we were in the crucial stage where the doctors were saying that there was not much they could do for me. Christmas 2009 was approaching and we said that these blood tests – which were basically different to those of a pathologist –

these were live blood cell tests where they look at the cellular make-up of the blood. They were in a mess, according to the naturopath, and I embarked on the approach he recommended and I could see improvement to the point now where yesterday I went to him for the first time for about four months and he said I was going really well. I've become his star pupil, because not too many people can handle the regime. Sue and I have, and I feel in excellent shape and I don't think I've got cancer any more.

The total package

The church has been a huge inspiration to have this direction in the back of my mind all the time. I think about a lot of things and I research and analyse a lot of things and I'm getting a lot of direction from the church and my involvement with God. I exercise a lot and I ride my bike to the support group to the point where quite a number of guys ask me what I'm doing. I've got a total of about 14 people talking to me from time to time getting input on what I'm doing. Only one of them so far has responded to the benefits of a spiritual approach. The rest are certainly switched on to looking at the naturopathic approach; some are even looking at meditation and relaxation – not many of them. I keep saying to them that it's the holistic approach that is everything: it's diet; it's exercise; it's belief; it's meditation; it's relaxation. All those things for me are important, and when people ask me what single thing can they do to improve their situation I say I don't know of any single thing. I think all these things are vital.

So, I've now beaten the Christmas 2010, the third prediction; the naturopath said yesterday that he was very happy with the way things were looking, and I'm feeling in great shape so I believe it's been a total journey.

Turning life around

I read a book when I first found out about the diagnosis where a lady said she was glad she got breast cancer because it was a journey that allowed her to turn her life around. When I read this, I thought, "Oh, this is garbage; who needs this sort of a journey". Four-and-a-half years down the track I now understand where she was coming from, and it is a journey and for those who want to take notice of what is presented to you in that journey I believe you can beat the problems. But it does take a very strong-minded person who had a belief and who believes in what they are doing.

I don't know of anybody in the support group who hangs in there and is dedicated to a diet regime. People do bits and pieces but not the lot; this is a bit too hard for most people. So, at the end of four-and-a-half years the blood tests are looking great; I'm feeling good; I have no pain; and the oncologist? He can get his business elsewhere as far as I'm concerned; I'm not going to the doctor's.

Thinking things through

Given that I've been a born-again Christian for about 14 months or so, I've had no serious downturn, but there have been a couple of times where I've been in a situation where I was thinking, "What do I do next?" So I won't say I get disappointed or lose faith, but it causes me to think long and hard about generally the situation I am in. But, because I am an analytical person, it's more of a thinking things through that causes me to write the pros and cons down about the particular thing I've been thinking about, so it causes me to think a little deeper but I can't say I've had any doubts most of the time during this. I can never say it's been a waste of time doing this.

Emotional involvement

I've been very emotional on each of the three times I have seen this Dr Mitchell – he's an evangelistic type of minister; he's been overseas a lot – to Pakistan and Czechoslovakia and other countries – and he's been gifted through God with the power of healing people. There have been some films on what he has done where people have had some serious health issue – people can't walk, are blind, things like this – and I'd say those times when I've been forward in the healing sessions and have had him "laying on of hands" for healing – when that's happened, that's when I've felt a heightened awareness, really, to the point where a couple of times I was a blubbering mess afterwards because the emotion was just so intense. Even now when I talk to people about it – I'm getting better at it – but when I first started explaining to people about it, I really had trouble trying to control my emotions when telling them. Yeah, it's really heightened at that time.

Everyday spirituality

I used to be a fairly hard-nosed person; at work I had a fairly responsible job and I used to say to people, "I don't get stressed, I give it". I had a lot of people working for me and a lot of union matters to attend to; I was in middle management. So I was in a mentally tough life. But I'd say that what's happened in the last 18 months is that I'm now much more forgiving about those things and I don't get involved in that sort of stuff anymore. So I'm calmer in myself; more placid. If someone wants to have an in-depth discussion that I don't agree with, I probably handle it more tactfully than I used to – it was "a spade was a spade and, if you want an argument, step right up". So I've certainly changed in that respect. Sue's noticed it and a few other people have noticed it, and I've had a couple of people say to me – knowing me from a long while ago – they couldn't believe that I'd changed to the point where I became a Christian; they never thought I would do that. I've become more relaxed in myself.

Focus in life – "to live as long as I can"

My purpose in life is now to live as long as I can, as healthy as I can, with a high quality of life. Sue and I have a great life together and I want to maximise that. I just don't want to be here for the years, I want to be in good health rather than be here and just breathing – there's no point in that, hence the intensity of exercising, relaxation, meditation, good diet, a belief in what I am doing, being a born-again Christian – all of that is just part of achieving the objective.

Personal spiritual support

There is spiritual support if I want it. On Wednesday nights we go to home group and there's usually about anything from 10 to 15 people there. It gets fairly personal from the point of view of being one on one. People talk about where they're coming from. I have had a couple of discussions individually with both pastors. It's here if I want it but in recent times I haven't felt any need for it; no problems at all. The guy who runs the first church we went to came from a very interesting background himself. He was involved in drugs and alcohol and had a tough earlier part of his life. He saw the light. He's a down-to-earth character who is totally different to a formal ministry, but his teachings from the Bible are given in a practical, down-to-earth, easy-to-understand way. So if I ever want to talk to him, there's no problem.

Meditating

Basically, I could never relax to the point where I could switch off entirely mentally. I don't need a lot of sleep, and Sue did yoga which, in the early stages, is meditation. I needed to get my mind in a more relaxed state. So I went along for a few weeks to meditation classes and came home and said to Sue, "I'm never going to get the hang of this". I was lying on my back there and I just couldn't get into it, couldn't switch off. Sue said, "Just hang in there, hang in there". After about a month, it started to click. Because I'm a goal- and objectives-setter and things like that, even though I'm not working, I still do that even though it's in a much smaller way than when I was working. So if I went to bed at night and I wasn't tired and my brain was still going, I've now developed a technique where I get out of bed and lie in a darkened room and I'll stretch and do relaxation and I do some meditation for probably about half or three-quarters of an hour. Usually I can go back to bed and go to sleep without too much trouble having done that.

I have a couple of forms of meditation. One is a routine where you breathe using a specific technique, and the other one is where you get your mind to concentrate, starting with your big toe, and go through your body parts and you try and communicate with your body parts – your toes, your ankles, leg, knees, hips right up to your head. I suppose some people say that's like counting sheep, but it does put your mind and body into a state where you are not thinking about what's going on from day to day.

Strong spiritual support

I've got plenty there – between the two churches and the two ministers. I have to say, too, that we've found some very nice people in the church we go to on Sundays. The church we go to on Wednesdays for healing is a much bigger church. A few people go to both churches so we've got contact with a few people more regularly, and there's much more of a family environment there but, no, I don't see any need to get any extra input or involvement.

Closer to people

I've found that I have become closer to people through greater friendliness. Two of the guys down there have issues. One bloke was separated later in life. Another guy has a few problems with pain and he is wanting to improve his quality of life from a health point of view, so there's a bit of dialogue going on there – back and forth, but me helping him really. They're interested in what Sue and I are doing and stuff like that. It's friendliness. What it's done for me is that I was very disappointed, and am still very disappointed, with the way the human race was going generally. When I see all the things people are doing through lack of direction and showing a lot of pent-up hate and things like that, I found it very hard to come across people that I felt were quality human beings and it was good to come across a bunch of people in these two locations where there is some hope, there is some good people who have a good outlook on life. Unfortunately, they're in the very small minority, not the majority. It's disappointing to see that. Many people, like myself, were rushing past this sort of life and it's not 'til a wake-up call occurs that people stop like I did and take a look at what's going on around them. And all this rushing around and work and squeezing everything I can in at the weekend and so on is fine, but there are some other things in life as well. So, is that age? Is it because I've had a wake-up call? I think it's probably both.

I've worked on a couple of the tables for the prostate cancer support group where they talk with people at seniors' meetings and marine shows and things like that, and what I've found is that a lot of those who have been identified with a prostate cancer problem put their whole existence in the hands of the doctors and they're looking for that magical outcome based on what the doctors are going to give them or suggest what they should do. I think they're falling well short of what the potential is for them to do. I think if they're relying on the doctors, they don't have much hope. The doctors have their place but it's just a small cog in the whole exercise.

A regime – exercise and diet

I exercise regularly. I ride a bike anything from 1¾ hours to 2¼ hours every second or third day. I do weights; when it's raining I have a static bike inside that I ride. Push-ups, sit-ups and crunches – that sort of thing. I found particularly that, as I learnt from a book I read from a guy who runs another support group, I found a technique that gave a better outcome for incontinence problems. (I'm not incontinent after four years.) So I have a very active, healthy exercise regime.

From a diet point of view, Sue and I are vegetarians bordering on vegan and this came about because of my exposure to the naturopath. While we ate well, we didn't eat much meat; very seldom ate fried food, didn't go to Maccas and that sort of thing, but we learnt that there was another step forward. So we basically have no sugar, dairy, meat, yeast, alcohol – and never did smoke – and we eat fresh food. If it comes out of the ground, we eat it. We are very much built around a vegetarian diet.

Spirituality for me …
It is a package. Sue and I had a set of circumstances that occurred after I was diagnosed – we had a boat in Sydney and we used to spend our weekdays on the boat and, whenever I went down on the weekends, we'd go home. I'd been retired a few years by then; I retired at 60. The boat was costly and the maintenance would have been very costly except I did all the maintenance myself. When the doctors had completed the operation and the radiation – that's when they said there's not much they could do for me – we started preparing for me not being around much longer. We thought that the last thing we wanted to do was sell the boat, but we decided that if I wasn't around there'd be no point in having it; it would be a huge burden and weight for Sue, so we sold it. There were a number of things that happened when we decided to change our direction. When we decided to sell the boat and house, it happened very quickly.

It wasn't until we were up here for quite a while, and family was up here as well, we started to go to the church; we sat down one night and thought that all the things that had happened might have been a coincidence – but they weren't. There were too many coincidences that had occurred in a short space of time for them to be coincidence. We were directed; but we didn't know it at the time. So that's why I say it's a holistic thing because we probably had about five or six things that occurred in a short space of time that got us to this point of the church and Christianity and getting to the naturopath. If we hadn't made that first move in Sydney, none of that would have happened. We were directed, but we didn't realise it.

Coping with stress

It was a journey unfolding. I didn't want to accept that. When I was first diagnosed, it was a huge crush for Sue and I, sitting in the doctor's office, to hear him say, "I'm sorry, you have cancer". You could have knocked me down with a feather. I felt, give me a brick wall – I want to bust it down – because this shouldn't have happened to me: I've led a good lifestyle; I've always been active and exercised; I've had a very positive mind. This cancer happens to other people, not me. Sue and I had only been married for about six months at that point, so that was a huge hit. But then, pretty quickly, I thought, hang on, I'm hearing this doctor and we've got to find out everything we can right now because this bloke's appointment time is not going to last long. So we started looking for what was the next step. So that was a pretty heavy time.

Then when the operation was done, they used the scatter gun around the prostate and pelvic area in the hope of killing any other cancer cells. So after this surgery and treatment – the second point in my journey where I was crushed – I thought, I'm strong-minded, I'll get over this real quick! The percentage of survival was low. When I was told that the operation didn't deliver the success they had hoped for, that was another big down-turn, big blow, but it made me even more determined that I was going to beat it. Then at the end of the radiation when the PSA dropped, I thought, "Beauty!" But then after treatment and the trial program my PSA started to double every 1.3 months, I thought, this is not looking good; I'd better get on to the hormone treatment. That was another big setback but I kept saying, "There's got to be a way, there's got to be a way!".

Suddenly, I finally came to terms with the real issue. I said to the doctors, "What do I have to do to fix the problem? I don't want to have to react to the problem after the event". Nobody in the medical profession could deliver that. So I thought that there had to be an answer somewhere else. So then the rest of the journey started to evolve. When I started to go to the naturopath and about that time started to go to the church, that's when I knew that I was going to win this; I'm going to beat it. I keep saying to Sue, "I know that when you are diagnosed with prostate cancer there are no symptoms, so what's to say there is no problem right now? I have no symptoms". When I recall the blood cell tests about 18 months ago that showed a pretty poor quality of my blood, and I look at it now and my general well-being I'm really "up there!", and I've got all those things that are left to do in my life.

Incredible partner support

I have to say that if I hadn't had Sue in my life I would never have beaten it because it's taken a huge effort on her part to throw it. She lived in Korea for a few years and she had a pretty good outlook on quality cooking and Asian cooking and things like that – she did a lot of good cooking, and, basically, she put it and all the condiments to one side and had to start from scratch. She did a huge amount of research and I wouldn't have gotten by without her. She's had a huge impact on me having a good result.

I now just intend to keep on with the way I am going. We were talking one day about wanting to spread the word and minister other people. I didn't really think about it until one of the guys said, "You're actually doing that through those who are ringing you up and wanting you to talk about what you are doing". I hadn't really thought about it that way. I was sitting one day having a haircut and the lady … and we had a chat and she started to embark on a more healthy lifestyle as a result of that chat. She said to me one day, "I have a friend of mine who has some serious health problems and she's wanting to look at a natural approach. Do you mind if I give her your number so she can give you a call?" I said, "No". Anyway, this lady rang me on two occasions and we chatted about quality of life and a healthy life. She didn't have a religious background at all. What I didn't realise around that time was that I was ministering to those who see what's happening in their lives and want to learn a bit more.

A note from the editor

I hope you have found some benefit from reading these stories. All the men indicated that they received benefit from telling them, and it was their hope that other men in a similar condition would be helped on their own journey. If you would like to communicate with me about your prostate cancer, please feel free to contact me through Facebook. I have been affected directly by cancer (not the prostate variety) and know a little of the experiences people have during a cancer journey. I would especially be pleased to hear from the partners of men with this illness. It is very much a shared experience.

Laurence Lepherd

www.ingramcontent.com/pod-product-compliance
Lightning Source LLC
Chambersburg PA
CBHW070603290526
45790CB00002B/753